WALK OFF WEIGHT

Other titles by Andrew Cate

Throw Out Your Scales - ABC Books
Ask The Fat Loss Coach (ebook)
Taste Testers For Weight Loss - Allen & Unwin
Gutbusters Low Fat Snacks And Sweets - Allen & Unwin
Slim, Trim & Tasty - JB Fairfax

WALK OFF WEIGHT

An 8-week food and exercise plan that gets results

ANDREW CATE

ABC
Books

Published by ABC Books for the
AUSTRALIAN BROADCASTING CORPORATION
GPO BOX 9994 Sydney NSW 2001

First published 2007
Reprinted February 2007
Reprinted July 2007 (twice)
Reprinted November 2007

National Library of Australia
Cataloguing in Publication entry
Cate, Andrew.
Walk off weight: the 8-week food and exercise plan
ISBN 978 0 7333 2046 0
1. Reducing exercises. 2. Reducing diets. I. Australian Broadcasting
Corporation. II. Title.
613.7

Cover and internal design by Wendy Farley, Anthouse
Typeset in 9 on 12pt Helvetica Neue Light
Printed in Hong Kong by Quality Printing

5

WARNING The information in this book is general in nature, and not intended
to replace medical advice. Consult your doctor, a sports-medicine professional,
podiatrist or physiotherapist if you have any concerns.

Table of Contents

Dedication

I would like to dedicate this book to the three wonderful women in my life. To my wife Robyn, for her unconditional love and support, and feedback on every page, chapter, idea and recipe trial I dish out to her. To Chloe, with the face of an angel, a smile that will break a thousand hearts, and a laugh that is so infectious, I couldn't imagine being a happier or prouder father. And to Brooklyn, our wonderful little baby girl who can make my day with a single, cheeky grin.

1

Introduction

...and the alarming study that made me write this book

THIS BOOK combines information about one of the most popular forms of exercise (walking) with the most popular of all health and fitness goals (losing weight). By giving you a planned exercise program and diet to follow, I hope to inform, guide and motivate you towards a healthier, happier, leaner future.

Just so you know a little bit about me, I am a personal trainer and fat-loss coach, and have over 15 years' experience in the health and fitness industry. I am university qualified, and have my own personal training studio on Sydney's Northern Beaches. I have worked closely with thousands of people, and seen people dramatically change their body shape, and their lives.

Each week I scan the internet for the latest information and research on food, fitness and fat loss. I try to seek out useful and practical information to pass on to my clients, or send out as part of my weekly email health tip. A few years ago, I came across an amazing study that initially made me question walking as a useful fat loss exercise. You see, I have seen some people get great results by walking, but I have also seen lots of people who don't seem to respond too well at all. The key findings from this study from the Centre for Disease Control and Prevention in Atlanta ring true for virtually anyone who has laced up a pair of walking shoes. The study said: *'Ninety-four per cent of people who exercise mainly by walking do not walk frequently enough or fast enough to gain real health benefits'*.

In many ways, this came as a shock to me. I had been recommending walking for many years as one of the best ways to lose fat and get fit. But was I wrong? Had I been leading people down the wrong path? It seems that giving people general advice on how they should 'walk more' is not really enough.

One of the main inspirations behind writing this book is to help walkers get more out of their activity. It's not walking that's the problem, but how it's done. With a little help from the aforementioned study, I have come up with 10 common mistakes walkers make, and how to overcome them to get results. You can read about them in Chapter 3.

The other inspiration behind this book is to share my weight loss secret. In my role as a personal trainer and fat loss coach, I am often asked: 'What's the best way to lose weight? What's the secret, the magic solution, the miracle cure?' When people start out with a personal trainer, they often expect some sort of magical ritual at high noon, a special food to cut out, a miracle soup to brew, or a few secret words that will motivate them for life.

But the answer I give them, and the secret to weight and fat loss that I have seen work for so many people, often draws a blank stare. It makes me realise that – sometimes – it's not really what people want to hear. Some people will continue to search elsewhere to find what they want to hear, and invest their hard-earned dollars on the promises of supplements, gadgets, or other programs. Many will succeed for a few weeks, and then move on to the next program, promise or pill.

My secret to weight loss is to help people discover that there is no secret. The answer is simple – eat sensibly, and find an exercise you enjoy – then do both for life. Surely it can't be that simple. In truth, it may sound simple, but it's not. Only a small percentage of our population actually do it. Our world makes it easy to find junk food, delivered to your car window or front door so you don't have to move a muscle. Sensible eating and regular activity are hard when you are constantly bombarded with mixed messages, fad diets and claims of the health benefits of low fat, low carb, low GI, high protein and high fibre. People get so overwhelmed they don't know where to start, and they even get so confused that they just don't bother. Our world celebrates laziness and overindulgence, yet condemns the effects when we become overweight.

But if there has ever been a type of exercise people can enjoy, and stick to – it's walking. Anyone can do it. From the very fit to the couch potato and beyond, virtually everyone can start a walking program.

For me, walking is a wonderful part of my life, professionally, personally and socially. I walk regularly with my personal training clients to push them a little harder or just to get off the exercise machines at my studio and get outside on a sunny day. My personal training clients often walk on the days they don't train with me to maximise their results, while the walking plan outlined in this book is part of the fat loss coaching program I have used extensively, and to great effect.

I walk regularly with my wonderful wife, whether it is on weekends, on holidays or just to spend time together. Our little girl, Chloe, has clocked up many hours in our baby harness, exercise stroller and baby backpack as we have ventured out on bush walks and picnics. As I write this introduction, I am training for an 8-day trek through the jungles of Papua New Guinea where, with 6 other Aussie battlers, I will take on the Kokoda Track.

My hope is that this book not only guides you through the process of losing weight and body fat, but also encourages you to make walking a part of your life. It's not just about pounding the pavement. There really is something magical about an activity you can enjoy with your children, partner, friends, family and family dog. What's more, you can enjoy it anywhere for the rest of your life as a way to prevent illness, boost your energy levels and increase your quality of life. It's a lot better than wasting time in front of the television.

Let's get started, and take that first step.

Andrew Cate

P.S. Do you have any questions?

If you have any questions, queries or concerns about the 8-week challenge, or anything about this book, why not send me an email? I am passionate about helping people get moving, get active and get results, and I would love to hear from you. If you want more advice on which program is best for you, if a certain recipe is suitable, or what to do if you are losing motivation, don't hesitate to email me. I'll do my best to get back to you ASAP. My email address is: acate@iprimus.com.au and my website address is www.andrewcate.com. While you're at it, don't forget to subscribe to my free weekly email health tip – the 'Better Body Update'. Topics include fat loss, fitness, nutrition, and motivation.

2

The wonder of walking

'You have two doctors – your right and left legs!'
– Hippocrates

What walking can do for you

Walking is a fantastic and diverse form of physical activity. It's an easy, accessible and enjoyable way to lose weight, get fit, reduce stress and boost your energy levels. It can be done almost anywhere, anytime, by anyone, and best of all – it's free. All you need are some comfortable clothes and a suitable pair of shoes. Because walking is an aerobic activity, it is very effective for weight and fat loss. Aerobic means with air, so your body uses oxygen (and in turn fat) as an energy source. Being a low impact exercise (walkers always have at least one foot on the ground), there is only a small chance of injury. It also means there is no pain or discomfort. That's why they say walkers smile, and runners snarl. Beyond the physical benefits, walking can open up new experiences and boost your mental wellbeing.

The benefits of regular walking

- Is suitable for all age groups and fitness levels
- Makes you lose weight and fat
- Lowers resting heart rate
- Improves muscle tone and strength
- Improves quality of sleep
- Increases energy levels
- Relieves stress and tension
- Lowers blood pressure
- Improves circulation
- Improves digestion
- Reduces the risk of osteoporosis

Science says – You won't walk alone

Walking is the most popular type of physical activity in Australia. Even though the rate of participation in physical activity is declining, there has been an increase in the number of people walking within all age groups.

The different types of walking

There are several different variations and styles of walking, all of which you can incorporate into your exercise routine over time as you gain fitness and confidence. There are different names for some of these techniques, but the focus should be on the unique benefits they offer. It's up to you to determine how challenging and effective you want walking to be. There really is a different walking style for everyone.

- **Strolling** – A light, casual pace that is slower than a typical walk. At this low level of intensity, you can normally talk comfortably without getting breathless. You are unlikely to sweat (depending on the outside temperature), and can just take in the scenery. This is more a relaxation technique than an exercise.

- **Incidental walking** – Incidental walking is the short bits of activity you accumulate over the course of the day, such as walking from the car to work, to the bank or around the house. The reduction in incidental movement is one of the leading contributors to the increasing rates of obesity around the industrialised world.

- **Moderate walking** – This is a planned, low intensity exercise walk where you can talk comfortably. Your breathing rate is slightly elevated and you might begin to sweat after about 10 minutes depending on the climate. This type of walking is ideal for beginners or the very overweight. As a rough guide, this is around 100 steps per minute.

- **Fast or brisk walking** – This is a planned, moderate intensity exercise walk where you can talk only briefly between breaths. Your breathing is rapid, and you will begin to sweat after 3 to 5 minutes. This type of walking is ideal for fat burning.

- **Power walking** – Power walking is an extension of fast walking, where you take a slightly bigger stride and exaggerate your arm swing. You actually drive the arms more vigorously both forwards and backwards, bending the elbow at 90 degrees to target muscles in the upper back. This helps to burn extra kilojoules and fat.

- **Race walking** – This is the type of walking you see at the Olympic Games. It combines endurance and technique to walk at high speeds, with competition ranging from social levels to the elite. Race walking requires technical skill, as the leg bearing the body's weight must be straight from the moment it comes into contact with the ground until it passes under your body. This leads to the characteristic 'waddle', and the associated dramas with warnings and disqualifications when race walkers break from the correct technique.

- **Weighted walking** – Some people like to carry weights while they walk by using dumbbells or wearing a weight belt, vest, backpack or ankle weights. This adds variety and increases the demands on your heart and muscles, helping you to burn more kilojoules over a given distance. However, there are some precautions you should take. Don't carry weights if they alter your posture or place stress on your joints. Dumbbells can cause shoulder problems in some people, while ankle weights should be avoided completely, as they can alter your balance.

- **Shopping centre or mall walking** – A number of shopping centres open their doors in the early hours for walkers. Some even provide a personal trainer to put you through your paces. This provides a varied, safe, indoor option for walkers who get the chance to work out and window shop at the same time. Just try not to be tempted by smells drifting around the bakery shops and cafés. Call your local centre to see what they offer.

- **Nordic walking, pole walking** – Using ski poles (either singular or in pairs) adds a whole new dimension to walking, and reduces the impact placed on your lower body. Developed by cross-country skiers to build their endurance and strength in the off season, Nordic walking helps you walk faster and burn more kilojoules while hardly even noticing the extra effort. The poles make walking more of a whole body workout, using more upper body and abdominal muscles than regular walking. They can also be helpful to people worried about balance and stability. The poles can be used on asphalt, sand or grass.

Science says – Kilojoule use is poles apart

Nordic walking has been shown to increase the amount of kilojoules you burn by up to 45 per cent when compared to regular walking. It also helps to increase your heart rate by 5 to 15 beats more per minute.

- **Shallow-water walking** – If you have access to a large, flat body of water, shallow-water walking is worth a try. Wade into water that's about knee deep and just start walking. Bring each knee up as high as you can, and swing your arms to help propel you. After a while, you'll feel the resistance of the water build up, making it hard going. This is a great cardiovascular workout, and can also help to tone your bottom and thighs. After just a few minutes, you'll know you've been exercising. You can also try ankle or waist deep-water for variety and to adjust the intensity.

- **Deep-water walking** – With this type of walking, most of your body is submerged. You perform an exaggerated arm swing and walking action wearing a flotation device or lifejacket. The vest allows your legs to move freely in the water, without contacting the bottom. Deep-water walking works your whole body and burns just as many kilojoules as running, without the jarring and stress on your joints. The higher you bring your knees, the more kilojoules you will burn, in addition to developing strength and endurance. To really up the intensity and burn even more kilojoules, you can try deep-water walking without a buoyancy vest.

- **Hill or stair walking** – One of the best ways to add intensity and maximise the kilojoules burned during your walks is to use hills and stairs. Many people avoid hills, but they are your best friend if your goal is to lose body fat and weight. Try to plan your walks around the steepest hills and longest flights of stairs in your area.

- **Bushwalking** – Bushwalking gives you the chance to enjoy outdoor tracks and cross-country paths in our wonderful wilderness. Whether you go hiking through our national parks or just trek through some local bushland, it's a great way to get close to nature, spend time with friends and family and burn off some kilojoules.

- **Pram/stroller walking** – New parents who want to exercise and spend time with their baby can take advantage of the wonderful exercise strollers available today. The tyres are inflated, so the baby gets a smooth ride, and Mum or Dad can really power along. It's a great way to get out of the house and burn extra kilojoules. As you get fitter, try pushing the stroller up a few hills to really up the intensity.

 Science says – Walking helps mums deal with postnatal depression

A recent study compared a group of mothers with postnatal depression who met to chat about their problems with another group who pushed their prams three times a week. After the study, the group who walked had a significantly greater level of improvement in symptoms.

- **Fun runs/walks** – Organised walks and fun runs are a great motivational opportunity for anyone who is striving to reduce body fat and weight. It gives you a goal to train for and an excuse to push yourself a little harder than normal. They are usually open to all ages and fitness levels, and provide drinks and medical support along the way. If you become a regular participant, you will then have a time to beat each year.

- **Walking groups/clubs** – Walking groups and clubs make exercise more social and friendly. You can be part of organised walks, events and holidays and enjoy the support and camaraderie from fellow walkers. It's a great way to get involved in a non-competitive activity that caters to all ages and fitness levels. When you investigate the clubs in your local area, check to see the typical group size, how tough the walks are, and if the time of day and the days of the week suit you. If there are no walking groups in your area, you could always form one of your own.

Walking surfaces

In addition to the different types of walking, there are different surfaces you can walk on. Surface type will have a strong influence on your enjoyment of walking, the amount of kilojoules you burn, and your risk of injury. Softer surfaces cushion your impact, but place more stress on your ankle. Harder surfaces reduce the risk of twisting your ankle, but place more stress on the shins and knees. All surfaces have their advantages and disadvantages, and it's important to consider your unique preferences, goals and injury history. In many cases, alternating different surfaces is a good way to add variety and prevent overuse injuries. While I encourage you to choose your favourite path (increasing the chances that you'll stay motivated), it helps to be informed of all your options.

- **Sand** – Loose sand significantly increases difficulty and kilojoules burned during walking. Every time your foot pushes off to propel you forward, the little bit of give in the sand forces your body and muscles to work harder to keep you moving. It also provides excellent cushioning if you have any significant knee problems. If you find it hard going, you can always move closer to the water where the sand is harder, although this will reduce the amount of kilojoules you burn. Soft sand walking tends to utilise your thighs, buttocks and calves a little more than regular walking. Just be careful of your ankles. If you are feeling super keen, try walking up sand hills.

- **Grass** – Grass is harder than sand, but much softer than concrete or asphalt, so your kilojoule use is slightly higher. Taking advantage of grass on golf courses, parks and sporting fields usually gives you a pretty safe, stable surface to walk on. Good grass cut to the right height is almost like walking on a pillow, which is ideal for anyone with knee, shin or ankle problems. Just keep a look out for the odd drain or sprinkler system. Be extra careful walking on uneven grass surfaces.

Science says – Avoid the risks

According to a recent study, improper surfaces are one of the leading causes of injuries in walkers and runners. The worst choice was said to be an irregular, gravelly shoulder of a road.

- **Concrete** – Concrete surfaces such as footpaths are flat, even and accessible, and they reduce your risk of getting tangled in traffic. But concrete is the hardest surface you can walk on, being approximately 10 times harder than asphalt. This means it has the strongest impact on your joints and muscles, and is not recommended for people with shin splints. If you have some good concrete paths in your area, make sure you wear good walking shoes with suitable cushioning.

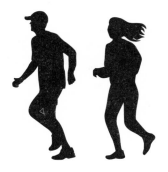

3

Walking to lose weight and fat

If you had to pick one activity that is best for weight loss, and suits the majority of people, walking is a clear stand out. To burn off stored fat, you have to burn off more energy (kilojoules) than you eat on a regular basis. With walking, there really is no cheaper, easier, and more enjoyable way to burn off kilojoules and body fat. But there are some important strategies to incorporate if you want to get serious results. Walking is actually a very easy, efficient activity for your body, so you need to do it regularly and quickly to get results.

10 common mistakes walkers make, and how to avoid them

As I mentioned in the introduction, up to 94 per cent of walkers don't walk frequently enough or fast enough to gain real health benefits. By applying a bit of knowledge, motivation and direction, together we can turn walking into the ultimate fat-burning exercise. Let's make it *you* who is one of the 6 per cent of walkers that not only gets real health benefits, but who achieves their health and fitness goals and gets great results. Following are the most common mistakes walkers make, and what you can to do avoid them in order to accelerate your weight and fat loss.

1 Not walking often enough

On one hand, it's a little hard to say how often you should walk, because it depends on your level of fitness, and the duration of your walks. But it's also important to spell out exactly what is required so you know exactly what it takes to get results.

- **For beginners** – Aim for 4 to 7 days a week. You need 1 to 2 months of regular walking to build a foundation of strength and fitness. After that, see below.

- **For weight loss** – Walking is a low impact, low intensity exercise, so you need to do it regularly to get results. If you are serious about fat and weight loss, or have serious amounts of fat to lose, you need to exercise every day. This might seem daunting, but don't let it discourage you. You can build up to it – and deep down, you must realise that doing very little now is probably not getting you results. Doing something every day boosts your metabolic rate every day, where you continue to burn kilojoules at a higher rate, even after your walk is finished. Your rate of fat loss will be more rapid if you can exercise this frequently. Do your best to exercise every day, or at least every other day. Don't miss walking two days in a row. You may even benefit from shorter walks in the morning and evening. Walking twice a day also helps to boost your metabolic rate.

- **For advanced walkers** – Aim for 3 to 5 walks a week. If you can walk very fast for 60 minutes, you should incorporate different activities into your program that challenge you. Try alternating days when you walk with other activities such as strength training, running, cycling or swimming.

2 Not walking fast enough

Speed matters. People who maintain a faster pace while walking will burn more kilojoules, and get better results. After a few weeks of regular walking, a leisurely stroll just won't cut it anymore. Some health authorities recommend people walk at a minimum speed of at least 5.6 kilometres per hour (3.5 mph). But using speed as a guide can be inaccurate, because it is harder for shorter people to walk at the same speed as taller people. Your speed will also vary depending on how fit you are, the duration of your walks, and if you are performing interval training.

For those reasons, I don't like to give out a specific speed you should aim for. But I will say you should walk like you're five minutes late. If your goal is weight and fat loss, faster walking equals faster results. If you really up your speed, you can get more benefit out of walking in the same amount of time. If you find it very difficult to walk fast over longer distances, use hills, and walk slower for a longer duration.

Science says – Take my breath away

If you can't hear your breath while you walk, you're not walking fast enough. Studies have shown that when you can hear yourself puffing during exercise, it's equivalent to working at approximately 65 per cent of your maximum heart rate. This heart rate zone is the minimum level required for burning fat as fuel during exercise. For beginners and those hoping to lose weight, light puffing is ideal. Really gasping for breath should be left to the advanced walkers, who would benefit from regular bursts of very fast walking or running to get breathless.

your level of effort

very helpful way to see if you are going fast enough during your walks is the rate of perceived exertion scale (RPE). This uses words on a scale of 0 to 10 to describe how hard you feel like you are pushing yourself at the time. It's easy to use, and is a fairly accurate guide to training at the right level to achieve your goals. The following chart comes in many forms, but the one below I have modified to help target weight and fat loss. As you can see, it's best to walk at a somewhat strong level (rating 5) for optimal fat burning, although beginners should take it a little easier (rating 2), and advanced walkers can go a little harder (rating 6). Get to know this scale, and bookmark it, as you will use it during your 8-week challenge.

Rating	Exertion level	Type of conditioning
0	Complete rest	No movement / elite couch potato
1	Extremely easy	Incidental movement
2	Very easy	Warm up / cool down
3	Somewhat easy	Mild fat burning / beginner
4	Moderate	Moderate fat burning
5	Somewhat strong	Good fat burning
6	Hard	Advanced fat burning / mild fitness
7	Very hard	Some fat burning / fitness training
8	Very, very hard	Good fitness training
9	Extremely hard	Advanced fitness training
10	Maximal	Sprints / elite fitness training

3 Not walking for long enough

While any exercise is better than none, you will need to walk for more than 10 minutes a day if you want life-changing, body shape-changing results. It's also important to consider how often and how fast you walk when determining how long you should walk for. One good way to work out the ideal duration is from a 7-day perspective, where you can vary your duration based on your frequency. Every 7 days, try to accumulate approximately 4 hours, or 240 minutes of walking.

4 x 60 minute walks per week
5 x 50 minute walks per week
6 x 40 minute walks per week
7 x 35 minute walks per week

When you are just starting out, any walking is ideal. Even short bouts of walking accumulated over the day can be beneficial, although you will have to motivate yourself to exercise more than once day. As you get fitter, longer walks will help to burn higher levels of stored fat. This is because blood sugars are prone to run out, leaving muscles with no alternative than to use fats as their energy source. As fitness increases over time, the body becomes more efficient at burning fat.

Science says – Short walks need to be fast

A recent study showed that short walks (15 minutes) do not burn off enough daily kilojoules to compensate for the yearly weight gain seen in many overweight people. The duration should be closer to 60 minutes for slow walking and 30 minutes for brisk walking.

4 Avoiding interval training, and slowing down on the hills

So many people walk at the same, steady pace, day after day, walk after walk. I even see people avoid hills on their walks, or slow to a crawl. But they are denying themselves the many benefits of interval training. Little random bursts of effort at different intensities really boosts the kilojoule-burning, fat-burning and fitness-increasing benefits of walking. For this reason, hills are a walker's best friend. They help you increase the intensity of your walks without having to go fast, or rely on running. Actively seek out hills and power up them. Think positively about hills, and view them as a short cut to getting results. Another great way to add intensity without impact is to use flights of stairs. This is also ideal if you live in a flat area. The chart below shows how hills and stairs can really ramp up your kilojoule use.

Exercise	Speed	Duration	Kilojoules	Calories
Walking	4 km/hr	30 min	415	99
Walking	5.5 km/hr	30 min	560	133
Walking uphill	5.5 km/hr	30 min	836	199
Stair walking	5.5 km/hr	30 min	1110	264

5 Not swinging your arms enough

Swinging your arms energetically can help you to burn up to 10 per cent more kilojoules while you walk. Swinging your arms a little faster will also encourage your legs to come along for the ride, and is a good way to increase your pace. Most people swing their arms, but it's the more pronounced, purposeful swinging that helps burn those extra kilojoules. Read Chapter 4 on walking techniques to help get your arms moving in the right direction.

6 Not adding variety

There's no doubt that variety is the spice of life, and the same rule applies to walking. If you stick to the same routine all the time, it's only natural that you will get bored, and find it harder to motivate yourself. Try to vary the location, time of day, intensity and duration of your walks to maintain interest. Look for ways to add variety to your walking routine.

How to vary your walking routine

- Use different types of walking
- Train for an event or fun run
- Walk on different surfaces
- Try interval training
- Try cross training
- Walk on a treadmill
- Walk with a partner or pet
- Use gadgets like a heart rate monitor or pedometer

7 Not walking faster as you get fitter, or measuring your progress

After walking for a few weeks, you will start to find it more comfortable as your leg strength improves and your lungs breathe a little more easily. The fitter you get, the more efficient your body gets at moving you around. This also means you will burn fewer kilojoules. Unless you continue to progress, and up the duration, intensity or frequency of your walks, your results will grind to a halt. So don't just plod along with your walks, otherwise you won't know how far you've come, or if you need to push things a little further. Keep a record of any information you can, such as the distance you cover, your personal best time over a given course, the intensity of your walks, the total duration of your walks or the total steps taken each day, week or month. Having times to beat or distances to cover also adds to your motivation. By completing the 8-week challenge in Chapter 7, you will learn how to use an activity journal. You will then have a tangible record of your progress, and a mark for you to improve upon if you want your results to continue.

Science says – Losing weight makes you burn fewer kilojoules

After initially walking on a treadmill and having their kilojoule use measured, an overweight group lost 20 per cent of their body weight through dieting over 12 months. Their kilojoule use was then re-measured at the same speed and distance on the treadmill. After losing weight, they used a staggering 35 per cent fewer kilojoules. In a similar study where obese males lost 21% of their body weight, the subjects exercised while carrying a backpack that weighed an equivalent amount to the weight they had lost. They still used 9 per cent less energy for the same walk. Their fitter, stronger bodies were more efficient.

8 Eating the wrong foods – drinking the wrong drinks

Whether you are concerned about weight control, fuelling your new walking program, or just maximising your health and vitality, what you eat and drink will have a massive impact on your results. Exercise is only half the picture. Don't just focus on your walking program, because if your diet is not up to scratch, you will struggle to lose weight. If you are going to invest the time and effort in an exercise program to burn off kilojoules, don't just add excess kilojoules straight back into your body. Fuel your walks with wholesome food that gives you energy, and actually helps burn fat. At the same time, cut back on high-kilojoule, low-nutrient foods and drinks that clog your fat cells. In the chapters that follow, you will find my full list of 10 fat-burning power foods to eat more of (with recipes), and the 10 fat-storing foods I encourage you to eat less of.

Science says – Don't just focus on one piece of the puzzle

A combined approach of healthy eating and regular exercise such as walking is scientifically proven to be the most effective method of long-term weight control. Don't just focus on one factor, and ignore the other.

alking before breakfast

ungry, your body is craving food, because its stored blood sugar els are running low. This is where your body is at when you wake up every morning. If you go for a walk when you first wake up (and your blood sugars are low), you are more likely to use stored fat as fuel. You don't necessarily burn more kilojoules, but you burn off a higher proportion of fat as fuel than someone who walks after breakfast. The difference isn't massive, but if mobilising and burning off stored fat is your goal – it all helps. There is also an argument that exercise on an empty stomach deprives you of energy, and you can't put enough effort into your walks. This may be true of elite athletes, people who exercise for more than 90 minutes, and possibly even advanced walkers, but it will help people aiming to reduce body fat. Some people can't exercise on an empty stomach, because they have diabetes, or because it just doesn't feel comfortable. That's fine. But if you get the chance, walk before breakfast a few days a week, or at least when you are hungry.

Science says – Exercise in a fasted state

Research shows that in a fasted state, up to 50 per cent more fat is used during cardiovascular exercise compared to people doing an identical amount of exercise in a fed state.

10 Avoiding weights

Unfortunately, there are many myths and misconceptions about lifting weights. What's worse is that the people who would benefit most (women over 40) are least likely to do it. As you get older, you naturally lose muscle tissue, which reduces your strength and energy levels, which results in middle-aged spread. Lifting weights can reverse this process – walking can't. Walking is a wonderful exercise, but it does very little to strengthen your upper body, or your abdominal core. Lifting weights also helps to protect your muscle tissue when you reduce your kilojoule intake, boosting your metabolic rate and helping with weight and fat loss. In addition, women get great benefits out of strength training, because they naturally have less muscle tissue than men. It's also more effective than walking at preventing osteoporosis. I don't suggest lifting weights instead of walking, but it's a great addition to any walker's health and fitness routine. Once you complete the 8-week challenge, why not give it a try?

Trainer's notes – Weights won't bulk you up

Don't worry about getting big muscles from lifting weights. That's probably the greatest health and fitness myth of all. As a personal trainer who has trained thousands of people, I have seen very few people get bigger from lifting weights. They all get firmer, stronger and feel better, but very few get bigger. Some men have the genetic potential to bulk up, but still need to dedicate their lives to it, eat like a horse and lift extremely heavy weights. But that's not the type of lifting I am encouraging you to do. Get advice from a personal trainer or exercise specialist if you have any concerns about starting a strength training program. You can also read a little more about lifting weights in Chapter 9.

10 barriers to weight-loss success

While overcoming the common mistakes that walkers make will boost your chances of losing weight, there are some other important barriers that you will need to conquer. Here are ten of the most common hurdles to weight-loss success, and how to overcome them.

1 High expectations

If you expect dramatic results, you should also expect disappointment. Slow and steady doesn't sound exciting, but it's the healthy way, the effective way and the only way that works long term. Focus on your direction, not your speed. Don't look for instant gratification. Focus on the process, and the results will come. The benefits from exercise and healthy eating come in weeks and months, not in minutes. Expect slow, gradual results from slow, gradual changes. Don't get frustrated if your progress is slow. The average Australian is gaining 1.7 grams of weight a day. If your weight stays the same for a month or two, you are succeeding.

2 Using weight as your only measure of success

I devoted a whole chapter in my last book to the problems with weighing yourself. Total body weight is often a poor indicator of fat loss, because you can lose fat but gain weight, and also gain fat but lose weight. This is because of the changes in muscle tissue that occur during exercise and strict dieting. I realise people like to see the scales come down, and they will, but don't weigh yourself all the time. Once a month is more than enough. Use other indicators such as waist circumference to measure your success. I have included a table in Chapter 7 where you measure a range of factors that can be improved with healthy eating and regular walking. It's also important not to forget the little things you can't measure, such as how you feel, what you've learned, and the improvement in your energy levels.

3 Lack of time

Everyone is busy, but we all have the same amount of time. The real issue here is priority. You will have to find a way to manage your time and yourself if you want to get results. Try to schedule your walks first thing in the morning, so there are less likely to be interruptions or reasons for you to put it off. Plan your meals in advance so you only need one trip to the shops. Learn to say no, and prioritise yourself. The best partner, parent, employee and friend you can be is a healthy, energetic one. The time you invest in walking will pay itself back many times over by improving the quality and quantity of your life.

4 Watching too much television

One way to find the time for walking is to cut back on the things that take up your time. The average person watches around 22 hours of television a week, so by substituting some of that time for walking, you can make a massive difference to your body shape. Television adversely affects your weight-loss potential, because it is an inactive use of time, you are more likely to snack while watching, and the types of snacks are more likely to be junk because of the influence of the advertisements you see.

5 You fall away on the weekend

Do you have a pretty healthy routine during the week, only to blow it all away by eating and drinking to excess on Friday and Saturday night? If that's you in a nutshell – you're not alone. One big weekend of over-indulgence and under-exercising can really put you behind the eight ball. You can still enjoy yourself, but why not try to minimise the damage. Take advantage of your break from work and be more active. Play some tennis, go for a walk, play with your kids, or do some vigorous gardening. You can also use the weekend to prepare for the busy week ahead, and pre-make batches of healthy food for freezing.

Science says – The weekend couch potato

Recent studies have shown that most people tend to take in more kilojoules on Fridays, Saturdays and Sundays. As the week rolls on, the subjects ate less fruit, while increasing their intake of take-away food and alcohol.

6 Special occasions

Is your diet always healthy, except for this one special occasion? I only drink more than a couple when I'm out with friends, or I only have dessert if my partner is having it, or I have to eat some cake for my co-worker's birthday. You might just make some huge inroads towards your weight-loss goals when you realise that these exceptions are more than a small distraction. Don't use special occasions as an excuse. From my experience, it's easy to find a special occasion if you want one. They just keep on coming. Try to foster a mindset where you can enjoy special occasions without large portions of unhealthy foods.

7 Not getting enough sleep

Studies have shown there is an important relationship between sleep and metabolic hormones, and that people who sleep less tend to eat more. Lack of sleep can raise the level of hormones linked with appetite and eating behaviour, making the sleep deprived more likely to gain weight. Staying out late on Friday or Saturday, then sleeping in the next day, is like triggering mini jet lag, and is a possible cause of Monday-itis. The other problem with lack of sleep is that you feel tired and fatigued, making it harder to motivate yourself to exercise. Try to make sleep a priority.

8 Not asking for help

Weight loss is hard enough at the best of times, especially when you go it alone. But there are many services available that can make things easier. Dieticians can help you to design a healthy eating plan, while an exercise physiologist or personal trainer can help you with your exercise program. Weight loss classes and programs enlist group support, while a fat loss coach takes a combined approach, working on your food, exercise and motivation to maximise your chances of getting results. If you are worried about the cost, drink a few less soft drinks and coffees each week, make your own lunch, ditch the magazines and stop smoking. Not only will you have more money in your pocket to afford professional services, your health will benefit as well.

9 The dieting mentality

If you think that the food changes you make puts you on a diet, then you are telling yourself you want to eventually get off the diet. This is especially true on strict diets, crazy rule diets (like only eat fruit when the sun is out) or 14-day detox diets. Any weight you lose will come back as soon as you return to your old eating habits. This type of dieting mentality is bad for your physical and mental health. It just doesn't work. Make slow, gradual changes you can stick to, and train your taste buds to enjoy healthy eating for life.

10 Motivation to change

There are different types of motivation that encourage someone to make changes. If that motivation is external, such as a nagging partner, it is much harder to stay on track. People who have external motivation often become experts at making excuses, because they are doing it for someone else. People who are internally motivated tend to find solutions when faced with a challenge, because they are goal driven and motivated from within. To switch on that internal drive, think long and hard about why you would like to change, and what will happen if you don't.

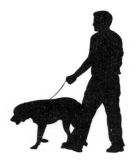

4

Walk this way –
top technique tips

10 tips towards terrific technique

Even though you have been walking since you were a toddler, it's still worthwhile to look closer at your exercise walking technique. For beginners, it is all about learning good habits from the start. For weight and fat loss, I want to maximise your chances of walking effectively and enjoying your walking. Even advanced walkers will benefit from reviewing their technique. Getting your stride, pace and posture right will not only help to reduce your risk of injury, but it maximises your chances of getting results. Following are 10 tips to make sure you start off on the right foot.

1 Perfect your posture

How you carry your body is important for preventing injury, and making your walking more comfortable. The two vital points on posture are to look forward, and stand tall. By keeping your head up, and not looking towards the ground, your airways will be open, allowing your lungs to breathe naturally. To protect your back, stand straight and tall with your shoulders back, your chest out, chin up and head high. Tuck your buttocks in slightly, which can help to prevent you from arching your back, or leaning too far forward.

2 Be aware of your core

Core strength is a real buzzword in health and fitness, and for good reason. Your 'core' is a general term used to describe a group of deep muscles in your abdomen, back and pelvic region. The core is a link between your upper and lower extremities, and the stronger your core, the more efficient and reliable the transfer of energy through the centre of your body. The core muscles support your spine, and a strong core adds stability and balance during walking. It will also help to improve your posture and pelvic alignment, making your movement more efficient, and reducing the stress on your lower back. A strong and stable core will help you stand straighter, breathe easier and even have more energy during your walks. If your core muscles are weak, then posture and movement can be compromised, resulting in back pain.

3 Activate your core

To utilise your core, you need to consciously contract your abdominal muscles, sucking your belly button into your spine. This is called 'engaging' or 'activating' your core, and is something that may take a little time to get used to. Start out by activating your core muscles while stationary, and then try activating your core muscles while walking. You can further strengthen your core with Pilates, yoga, Tai Chi and fitball classes. Over time, core activation will become more of a habit, and you will enjoy all the benefits that a stronger core has to offer.

 Science says – The benefits of being strong to the core

Recent research suggests that strengthening your core muscles will help to improve your athletic performance and prevent injuries. For optimal results, perform core-strengthening exercises at least 2 to 3 times a week for 15 to 20 minutes.

4 Swing your arms

Swing your arms freely in time with your feet, keeping your elbows bent to a 90 degree angle and drive them to the rear. Your shoulders should stay down and relaxed, while your fingers should be loose and partially curled inwards. Don't swing your arms with your elbows straight, and avoid clenching your fists, which can raise blood pressure levels. The front hand shouldn't go past the centre point of your body as it comes up from your side. Strong swinging is okay, but exaggerated pumping and raising your arms too high won't propel you any faster, and can stress your shoulder.

5 Roll your foot from heel to toe

With each step, your heel should touch the ground first. This foot then takes all your weight until the other heel strikes the ground. After the initial contact, smoothly roll your foot from heel to toe, or more precisely, to the ball of your foot. Try to flow forward, and avoid marching, crashing or slapping your feet into the ground. This helps to minimise the stress on your ankles, knees, calves and shins. Rolling through your step helps you get a good push off, and powers you to walk faster.

6 Push forward with your back foot

When you start to stride out, push yourself forward off the ball of your back foot. The stride length behind your body should be longer than out in front, as your front leg provides no power. Aim for more frequent smaller steps rather than taking longer steps to increase your speed. It's also important to propel yourself strictly forwards instead of vertically. If your body bounces up and down rather than forwards, the impact on your foot is increased.

7 Be aware of your breathing

It's easy to forget about the importance of breathing during exercise, but it can make a difference to your rhythm, and results. During exercise, we naturally increase the rate, not the depth of our breath. You will notice this after a few minutes of steady walking. It is oxygen that fuels fat burning during exercise, so make sure you are taking in enough. Timing your breath with each step, and breathing a little deeper, can help supply oxygen more efficiently. Ideally, your body will naturally exhale when each foot touches the ground, creating a breathing cycle, otherwise known as rhythmic breathing. Timing your breathing in this way improves airflow to the lungs, and even helps support the spine to absorb the impact of each step. Trying to breathe a little deeper while you walk will also help to oxygenate your blood more completely. If you exhale more completely, it's easier to take a deeper breath. Breathing deeply also helps you to unwind and relax during your walks.

 Science says – Belly fat inhibits breathing

Fat stored around your stomach is more responsible for shortness of breath during exercise than overall body fat or lung function. People with higher levels of abdominal fat need more oxygen during exercise.

8 Adjust for slopes

A change in gradient should bring about a subtle change in technique. When walking uphill, lean forward a fraction, and put more energy into swinging your arms. This helps you to power up the hill without stressing your back. When walking downhill, it's also important to adjust your technique, as it places more stress on your knees. Try to maintain a comfortable, if not slightly slower speed, and take shorter steps. Bend your knees a little more and plant your feet gently, which helps to cushion the impact.

9 Be relaxed

If you are going to modify your technique, make one change at a time. People trying to change too many things at once can appear stiff, and find it hard to walk naturally. Walk smoothly and relax your neck, shoulders and back, keeping your hands loose and unclenched.

10 Avoid the common mistakes

Walk correctly, and you're on the right path to weight loss, weight control, good health and vitality. Walk incorrectly, and you are on the fast track to injury, inactivity and de-motivation. Following are four of the most common mistakes walkers make with their technique, and how to avoid them.

- **Don't chicken walk** – Avoid walking with your elbows out to the side. Keep your arms and elbows close to your body.

- **Avoid long steps** – Although I want to encourage you to walk fast, make sure you do it with more frequent steps rather than longer steps. This can place unnecessary stress on your shins.

- **Don't look down** – Looking down and staring at your feet tilts your head down, which affects your posture and breathing. Look up and enjoy the view.

- **Throw out your old shoes** – Shoes that are not designed for walking, that fit you incorrectly, or that have lost their cushioning after 6–12 months of use can do more harm than good.

The correct walking technique checklist

- Look straight ahead, not down
- Breathe deeply and steadily
- Pump your arms and bend your elbows at 90 degrees
- Keep your tummy and your buttocks tucked in
- Step onto your heel, roll through to the ball of your foot
- Push forwards off your back toes

5

Shoes, clothes and accessories

10 tips to choosing the right walking shoes

The one essential piece of equipment you will need for walking is a good pair of shoes. It's the only real expense that's necessary for walking, so for the sake of your feet, try not to cut corners on your shoe budget. Footwear that is correctly fitted and designed specifically for your activity can add comfort and prevent injury. On the other hand, inappropriate, ill-fitting or worn-out shoes can cause blisters, corns, calluses and foot problems such as heel and arch pain, stress fractures and Achilles tendonitis. Choosing the right pair of shoes can be confusing and complicated if you don't know what you're looking for. Keep the information in this chapter close at hand to help evaluate your current pair of shoes or select a new pair.

1 Ignore the brand and colour

Good fit, support, and cushioning are more important than appearance, popularity or celebrity endorsements. The manufacturing standards of most major shoes companies have improved dramatically in recent years, with a lot of work going into the development and design of shoes specifically suited to walking. Some brands will just suit people's feet more than others, so don't get too caught up in their reputation.

2 Buy walking shoes

If you intend to start a walking program, you need to get walking shoes. No single pair of shoes is right for all activities. There really is a difference between walking shoes, aerobic shoes, and cross trainers. Old-fashioned sneakers are not good for walking. Shoes that are specifically designed for walking are best at reducing the unique stresses and forces placed on your foot during every step. Because walking predominantly involves forward motion, walking shoes provide front-to-back cushioning, unlike sports shoes that have more lateral support. If you walk very fast, or like to do a little bit of running during your walks, running shoes will be suitable. They will be much better for your feet than a flat pair of tennis shoes.

3 Seek out a soft landing

Walking can put up to 100 tonnes of stress through your feet during an average 60-minute workout. That's why it's important to purchase shoes that give your feet adequate cushioning, especially if you walk on hard surfaces. Look for shock-absorbent soles and good padding in the heels. Jump up and down in the shoes when you try them on. Well-cushioned shoes will give you a soft landing.

4 Heel support is vital

The structure at the back of the shoe that cups your heel should be firm, and fit snugly. There should be no slippage at the heel, and your foot should feel stable from side to side. It should be broad enough to provide a stable platform for your entire foot. Your heel should be held in the shoe, and supported somewhat higher than the rest of your foot. Make sure the top back of the shoe doesn't rub hard against your Achilles tendon. Many shoes have what's called an 'Achilles notch' to prevent this problem.

5 Look for flexibility

After striking the ground heel first, the foot rolls gradually from the heel to your toes. That's why walking shoes should be flexible from the heel to the toe to match the movement of your foot as it rolls through each step. A walker's forefoot flexes nearly twice as much as a runner's, especially if you are walking fast. The shoe should bend at the toe area, and also twist a little from side to side. Walking shoes should not feel stiff as a plank, or restrict foot flexion.

6 Find a comfortable fit

Walking shoes should feel comfortable in the store. Do the laces up properly and walk around in them to ensure they fit properly. When standing, the gap between your longest toe and the front of the shoe should be about equal to your thumbnail (roughly 15 mm). They should feel light-weight and breathable. If they feel comfortable immediately, that's a good sign. The shoe should feel snug and firm, but roomy enough so you can wiggle your toes. You shouldn't be able to wobble in the shoe when you rock from side to side, and from front to back though. If your forefoot bulges over the side, they may be too tight. The shoe shouldn't need to be stretched, or broken in. If the shoes feel a little tight, don't buy them. Your feet swell when you walk for 30 minutes or more, so you may need a size larger than your dress shoes.

7 Know your feet

There is no 'best' walking shoe on the market because everybody's feet are different, and people have different walking styles. Get to know any special requirements your feet have. For example, people with high-arched feet usually need more cushioning and lateral support than those with average feet. On the other hand, people with flat feet need more arch support and heel control. If you have weak ankles that tend to roll or sprain easily, lateral stability will be a priority. Some people have one foot bigger than the other, and others have wide or narrow feet. After you have been through a few pairs, you will get to know what features and brands suit your needs best. If you have any special concerns, it may help to see a podiatrist, who can assess your feet, and recommend the best shoes for you. They may look at your gait, stride, weight distribution and even look at your old shoes to detect any problems. This is essential if you have any knee or ankle problems, or if you over-pronate (roll too far inwards) or under-pronate (don't roll enough).

8 Ask for help when shoe shopping

Specialty stores generally have a wide selection of shoes with different styles, sizes, lengths and widths. They also should have staff trained to help you select the best shoe based on your activity and the anatomy of your foot. Foot size and width can actually change a little as you get older, so it doesn't hurt to have your feet measured before trying on shoes. It may also help to enquire about different lacing techniques. There are a number of ways you can lace your shoes to help take pressure off certain areas and support others. This can be especially helpful if you have narrow feet, wide feet, foot pain, high arches, corns or an in-grown toenail.

Science says – Get the right size Cinderella

A recent study found that 88 per cent of women wear shoes too small for their feet. It's believed that the social pressure to have small, dainty feet is behind the problem. This can cause foot, ankle or even knee problems down the track.

9 Replace worn shoes

Shoe wear depends upon on your foot anatomy, body weight, type of exercise, frequency of training and the training surface. If you use them regularly, most shoes will lose their cushioning within six to twelve months, which can place the jarring back onto your knees and ankles. Don't wait till your shoes have holes in them before buying another pair. To prolong their life, wear your walking shoes only for your workouts, rotate between two pairs so they can 'bounce back' between walks, and replace your inner soles occasionally to maintain cushioning.

10 Final considerations for shoe shopping

- Buy shoes in the afternoon, or after you have been walking around for a while, when your foot size is at its maximum.
- When trying on shoes, be sure to wear the same socks you will be wearing during your walks.
- Try on both shoes. Many people have one foot larger than the other. If one foot is larger than the other, buy the larger size.
- Sizes vary among brands and styles, so pick shoes based on how they fit your feet.
- Don't shop for shoes when you are in a hurry. Walk around in the shoes after trying them on.
- Try on more than one pair so you have something to compare.
- Experiment with the narrow and wide lacing eyelets to help custom fit the shoes to your feet.

Get dressed for success

Don't get caught with your socks off

The right socks can help to prevent blisters, and make your walks just that little more comfortable. The correct fit is important, because a tight fit can become constricting, while too loose, and they bunch up, causing pressure points, shearing forces and blisters. Good quality socks are also made of fabrics designed to draw sweat away from the skin on your foot. Keeping your feet dry helps to prevent odour and blisters, especially if you are a person whose feet sweat heavily. The sock needs to be shaped like your foot to keep the sock snug and prevent bunching. Some designs also use elastic to keep them in place, while others have extra padding or extra stitching across the toe and heel for strength. Experiment with different brands to find the style and features that suit your feet the most. Avoid cotton socks, tube socks and socks that are not gender specific, as men and women's feet have a different shape.

Some good ideas about your gear

The most important thing about what you wear, no matter what pace you walk at, is to feel comfortable. Ideally, you want to be totally unaware of what you have on so you can put everything into your walk. If you are walking at a slow to moderate pace, loose fitting clothes will feel fine. As your fitness level and speed increases, you may find tighter fitting clothes more appealing, which don't rub or flop around. Walking outside is a year-round activity, but there are also special considerations you might need to take depending on the climate and time of day.

Clothing for cold and wet conditions

The wind and rain shouldn't stop you from walking. Skin is waterproof. Improvements in fabric technology and design mean you can keep warm and dry in most conditions. Dress so you can remove layers as you warm up after a few minutes, and put them back on as you cool down. You may need to carry a small back pack, or tie clothes with long sleeves around your waist. Really cold temperatures might also require a thermal under-layer, gloves and a ski mask. Synthetic fabrics trap layers of warm air, absorb sweat and keep moisture away from your skin to prevent you becoming wet and chilled. It is estimated that a third of your body heat is lost through the head, so wear a hat or beanie if it's really cold. A vest can be good, as it keeps your trunk warm but allows you to swing your arms freely. A set of waterproof pants, a jacket and gloves may also be a good investment depending on your climate.

Clothing for hot weather

When it's hot, try to wear light, loose-fitting clothing, and avoid tight-fitting shirts and sweat pants that cause perspiration and fluid loss. Try to look for thinner socks, light T-shirts and comfortable walking shorts. Some clothes are also manufactured to make life more comfortable for people who sweat profusely, which is more of an issue in the heat. It will also be advisable to wear a hat or cap, and sunglasses to protect your eyes. See Chapter 12 for more information on walking in the heat.

Walking accessories and toys

There is a wide range of gadgets and workout toys available to make your walking routine more interesting. To help keep your hands free and your arms swinging, most of these items are small and light weight. They can range from tools to help monitor your progress, such as heart rate watches and pedometers, to fun devices like MP3 players that help keep you motivated. There are plenty of ways for you to accessorise your exercise. The options are really only limited by your budget and your imagination. Just remember, they won't do the work for you.

Pedometers

Pedometers are an inexpensive way to measure your distance travelled, kilojoules used and total steps taken during a walk. By attaching a pedometer to your belt or waistband, you've got a cheap, easy to use tracking device that keeps you motivated and informed. It's interesting to measure your total steps, and a good pedometer will give you a clear indication of how much activity you actually do, not what you think you do. Just wearing a pedometer increases your awareness of your daily activity and exercise levels. They are also a very effective way of measuring your incidental exercise, which is known to be an important factor in weight control. It recognises the little bits of movement you do throughout the day, such as taking the stairs instead of the elevator, or parking a little further from your destination. Once you work out the average amount of steps you take for a few days, challenge yourself to go higher, aiming to reach at least 10 000 steps a day.

Some interesting facts on steps

- 1 kilometre = 1200 average steps
- 1 mile = 2000 average steps
- 10 minutes of walking = 1200 average steps
- Minimum steps for weight loss (per day) = 12 000 average steps
- Minimum steps for weight loss (per week) = 80 000 average steps
- Typical office worker = 2000 to 3000 average steps per day

 ### Science says – Take the right amount of steps

It's recommended that you accumulate 12 000 steps per day, or around 80 000 steps per week, for significant weight and fat loss. This is equivalent to around 40 to 60 minutes of daily activity. These guidelines can be reduced a little if you are very overweight, and beginners should build up to these levels.

Heart rate monitors

Heart rate monitors can be a great addition to your walking routine. They allow you to continuously check your exercise intensity (heart rate), and make sure you are reaching the goal of a particular workout. They eliminate the guesswork from measuring your training intensity, allowing you to increase or decrease your training intensity to maximise your chances of burning kilojoules and fat. They usually have two parts, including a chest strap to sense your heartbeats, and a watch that displays the reading. Many models allow you to set training zones, which make a beeping sound if your heart rate strays from the desired performance level. See the section on 'Heart rate training' on page 144.

Satellite Navigation (SAT NAV) devices

Sounds complicated, and they aren't cheap, but if you like your workout toys, these devices are sensational. They strap onto your arm and give you all sorts of information about your walks, such as time, current speed, average speed, kilojoules burnt and distance walked. They are incredibly accurate and simple to use. Some models even allow you to download the data from your walks onto your computer so you can measure your progress. Some brands have models specifically designed for walkers.

MP3 players

If you like to walk alone, music is a great way to motivate yourself, and new technology has made music more portable than ever. MP3 players are lightweight, reasonably priced, and can store hundreds if not thousands of songs on a device not much bigger than a box of matches. Make sure your MP3 player is loaded with songs that inspire you to go fast and hard, and maybe some relaxing music for cool downs or longer strolls. Whatever style of music you prefer, just make sure it's not too loud, as you need to hear traffic noise to ensure your safety.

Body fat monitoring scales

Body fat monitoring scales allow you to measure your progress a little more accurately than just measuring your weight. After entering your age, gender and height, the scales send a harmless and undetectable electrical pulse through your body while weighing you. They then take all this information and calculate how much of your total body weight is body fat. If you are a beginner, or if you are performing strength training in conjunction with your walking program, these scales may be very helpful. This is because some of the weight loss (fat loss) that you obtain from walking will not reveal itself on normal scales, because an increase in muscle density (not bulk) will cause you to gain a little weight (not fat).

6

The Walk Off Weight diet plan

Let's end the confusion about food

In the time I have studied and read about nutrition, I have seen more conflicting information and heard more food myths than I care to remember. That's because nutrition is a rapidly changing field of science, with new studies altering our point of view on what seems like a daily basis. In addition, information on nutrition can vary depending on the person it is intended for. For example, fruit juice is ideal if you are an athlete, but detrimental if you are trying to lose weight and fat. There is no 'one diet for everyone'. What's more, fad diets, supplement companies and even food manufacturers play on this confusion to help sell their products. For example, high-fat fast meals get promoted as 'healthy' salads, and breakfast cereals devoid of fibre are promoted as low fat.

What foods help to fast track weight loss?

After fine-tuning my dietary recommendations for over 10 years with my personal training and fat-loss coaching clients, I have come up with 14 proven strategies for health, fitness, energy and weight loss. What's more, you'll be glad to know that the recipes and 'fast feast' ideas later in the book show you how to eat better without losing taste. Eating is an enjoyable part of life, and I don't want that to change for you. But if you can stick with this diet for 8 weeks, you will look better, feel healthier and want to make it your lifetime eating plan. That's because it tastes good, and it gets results.

14 food strategies that accelerate weight loss

1   Cut back on kilojoules
2   Get your portions under control, especially at night
3   Become a naturalist, and eat more natural food
4   Don't medicate yourself with food
5   Have a grease and oil change
6   Be patient, positive and prepared when changing your diet
7   Drink more water, less sugar
8   Forget the fads, celebrity diets and magic pills
9   Adjust your kilojoule intake for inactivity or indulgence

10   Don't snack if you're inactive
11   Always eat breakfast
12   Eat more food prepared at home
13   Don't beat yourself up if you indulge occasionally
14   Eat less fat-storing foods

Strategy 1 – Cut back on kilojoules

By eating too many kilojoules, and not burning off enough of them, people gain weight and body fat. To lose weight and body fat, you need to reverse the process by consuming fewer kilojoules and burning off more. Think about the high-kilojoule aspects of your diet (or keep a food diary) to identify the areas you can improve upon. You need to create a kilojoule deficit, so your body burns off not just the kilojoules you eat, but also the reserve of excess kilojoules stored on your body as fat. The key is to eat enough protein, and only cut back on your kilojoule intake gradually. Severe kilojoule restriction, or starvation, will only send your metabolism into 'shutdown'. Cutting back your kilojoules gradually protects your metabolism, helps you maintain existing muscle mass, and prevents hunger. Let's face it; the only way you will stick to dietary changes over the long term is if you enjoy them. Nobody can enjoy a diet where you have to go hungry.

Great ways to cut back your kilojoule intake

- Add extra vegetables to your meals
- Add chilli to your meals
- Drink water before your meals
- Cut back your alcohol intake, and have alcohol-free days
- If you must have fruit juice, water it down
- Use food labels, and choose the lowest kilojoule option
- Have lots of salads in summer, and soups in winter
- Spray cooking oil, don't pour it
- Measure your serving sizes once in a while to maintain awareness
- Have one low carbohydrate meal per day

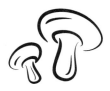

Science says – More protein with less kilojoules accelerates fat loss

Lower kilojoule diets that have a higher proportion of protein with fewer kilojoules from carbohydrates can accelerate fat loss faster than high carbohydrate diets of an equal kilojoule content. Studies have shown that lower carbohydrate/high-protein diets were twice as good at maintaining the body's metabolic rate, and also promoted greater feelings of fullness from an equivalent amount of food.

Strategy 2 – Get your portions under control, especially at night

Portion size is vital for weight control, because the smaller your serving, the smaller your kilojoule intake. Unfortunately, people have become accustomed to large serving sizes, and feel compelled to finish whatever is put on their plate. This translates to a lot of people consuming more food (and kilojoules) than their body needs, and those extra kilojoules are simply stored as body fat. The push to promote low-fat foods has also encouraged people to eat without guilt in the belief that anything without fat is open slather. But remember, you have to burn off what you eat, plus a little extra, to lose body fat and weight. It doesn't matter if the food is low fat, reduced fat or no fat, it still has kilojoules you have to burn off. Your metabolic or kilojoule-burning rate is slowest at night, so it's the meal you are least likely to burn off.

How to cut back on your portion sizes

- **Slow down** – Eat more slowly to get more fullness per mouthful.
- **Eat well** – Unprocessed foods such as legumes, fruits and vegetables are absorbed slowly, making you feel fuller for longer.
- **Drink water** – Water can help to suppress your appetite by keeping your stomach full, taking the edge off your hunger.
- **Eat less, more often** – Cut down on the amount of food you eat and have smaller meals more often.
- **Get familiar** – Familiarise yourself with a healthy portion size of the foods you eat most often.
- **The danger zone** – Enjoy but make sure you minimise your portion size of high-kilojoule foods such as biscuits, cakes, pastries, sweets, fats, oils, spreads and processed carbohydrates.
- **It's fair to share** – Share entrées and desserts when eating out at restaurants.

Science says – Beware of portion distortion

Studies show that we often eat too much and don't judge the size of our servings well. Most people eat more than the recommended serving sizes for many foods. It has been estimated that the average person consumes 600 kilojoules more every day than they did 20 years ago.

Strategy 3 – Become a naturalist, and eat more natural food

If you want results, if you want to shed fat, if you want to feel well and prevent disease, then healthy eating is a must. But unfortunately, our society seems to suffer from what has been termed a nature-deficit disorder. So much of our food is packaged, processed, puréed, powdered or preserved, delivered to your door or via your car window. This also means we get fewer nutrients, resulting in high-kilojoule foods with a reduced capacity to make us feel full. Fortunately, the solution is simple – use the fruit and vegetable section of your supermarket. It's packed with real, vibrant, high-nutrient foods ready to be eaten as nature intended. Generally, the closer a food is to its natural state, the better. A useful term is 'human interference' (HI). You will be much more likely to succeed at weight loss if you seek out foods with minimal HI, such as quality proteins (without fat), quality fats (plant fats) and quality carbohydrates (unprocessed). The more natural foods you eat, the less you will need to rely on junk food. It may take you a while to get the taste and passion for natural foods, but your success will depend on it.

Strategy 4 – Don't 'medicate' yourself with food

Feelings of sadness, anger, stress, exhaustion or frustration are a part of life, and how you deal with these emotions can have a big impact on your body shape. They can all lead to eating that is a little out of control, and detrimental to your health and weight. This is often termed emotional or comfort eating, where people use food to preoccupy themselves, or anaesthetise themselves against negative emotions. Food is used to regulate mood, cope with stress or overcome feelings of anxiety or boredom. Because the foods used to deal with negative emotions are usually unhealthy (alcohol, chocolate, chips, ice cream, cake), emotional eaters often find it hard to lose body fat. Over time, a very strong bond can form between certain foods and certain emotions. The food serves as a distraction from the problem, but it won't alleviate it.

Warning signs you are an emotional eater

- Eating when you're not hungry
- An urgent need to eat
- Eating when you're bored
- Fast eating
- Continuing to eat when you are full
- Getting a second serving without even realising
- Eating alone out of embarrassment at the large portions
- Eating alone out of embarrassment at the type of food consumed
- Eating until uncomfortably full
- Feelings of guilt or self-loathing after overeating
- Strong cravings for specific foods

How do you overcome emotional eating?

Occasional emotional eating is normal, however frequent emotional eating can become a serious problem. Don't wait for the problem to go away, or think you can eat your way out of it. The first step is to increase your awareness, and learn to recognise the difference between emotional hunger and physical hunger. Try to increase your awareness before and during eating, and try to examine what, how much and why you eat. Identify the events and feelings that are associated with your uncontrolled or emotional eating. Focus on the cause and solution, rather than automatically responding by eating. As you become more aware, you can begin to tackle the problem and disconnect food with your emotions. Stop using food as a comfort or reward. Try to find non-food related methods of coping with your emotions, such as exercise or relaxation strategies. Until you tackle the underlying issues that lead you towards comfort eating, sustained fat loss will be very difficult. In some cases, life coaching or counselling to help deal with the underlying emotional issues will be the best course of action.

Strategy 5 – Have a grease and oil change

Fat is extremely high in kilojoules, and it's important to cut back your intake to help lose body fat. But while high-fat eating is a nutritional disaster for weight and fat loss, fat-free eating doesn't necessarily work either. That's because all fats and oils are not created equally. When you do eat fats, try to cut back on the saturated fats and trans fats found in butter, full cream milk, junk foods, pastries, cakes, chicken skin, beef fat and processed meats. These types of fat are more likely to be stored in your fat cells, and less likely to be used as fuel once they're stored. They are also the most dangerous type of fat for your heart. Replace them with small amounts of natural, minimally processed fats such as those found in avocado, nuts and seeds, fish, flaxseed oil and extra virgin olive oil. A diet that contains 'moderate' amounts of healthy fats helps to curb your appetite, provides fuel that is more likely to be used than stored, and tastes better than a strict low-fat diet. It can also result in more weight loss over the long term. A moderate-fat diet is similar to that of Mediterranean people, who consume moderate amounts of nuts and unheated oils with salads, vegetables and breads.

Science says – Low fat is hard to stick to over the long term

In a study that compared a typical low-fat diet with a moderate-fat diet, people experienced roughly the same amount of weight loss after 6 months. But after 12 months, those who ate the moderate-fat diet lost about 4 kilograms more, while those on the low-fat diet regained their original weight, plus an extra 2.5 kilograms. The people consuming a moderate-fat diet stuck with their healthy eating plan, said foods were tastier, and consumed more of their favourite foods while watching their portion sizes.

Strategy 6 – Be patient, positive and prepared when changing your diet

Patient – Make sure you acknowledge that it takes time to change your diet. I encourage people to ease into healthy eating, because I know it takes time to train your taste buds. By making small changes and building on those gradually with additional small changes, you will create new habits. On the other hand, dramatic changes are hard to stick to, and usually lead to a dramatic bounce back to your old lifestyle.

Positive – If it takes time to change your diet, you are going to need a positive attitude. If you want to change your body shape, it will help to change your thinking. Obviously, it's normal to be struck down with negative thoughts now and then, but don't let it stop you reaching your goals. Tell yourself that you have the ability to make this happen, and focus on your small achievements along the way. Share your thoughts and goals with other positive people, and strive to find tasty, healthy recipes you enjoy.

Preparation – Getting organised with your food can make it a lot easier to eat healthily, and reduce your kilojoule intake. Put aside 15 minutes each week to plan your meals, and stick to your list when you go shopping. You will then have healthy foods on hand for breakfast, lunch, dinner and snacks, and be less likely to grab junk on the run. This strategy is especially helpful when you are first changing your diet.

Strategy 7 – Drink more water, less sugar

The amount of water you drink can have a massive impact on your health and body shape, especially if you drink it instead of kilojoule-laden drinks. Drinking kilojoules in any shape or form (with the possible exception of skim milk smoothies) is a good way to pack fat onto your body. Fruit juice, soft drink, alcohol, cordial and sports drinks are packed with extra kilojoules that won't fill you up, yet they need to be burnt off before you will access and remove stored kilojoules (body fat). One can of soft drink takes around 25–30 minutes of walking to burn off, and that's just to get you back to evens. You will need to do more to burn off existing stores of body fat. If you can't go without these drinks, water them down, and wean yourself off them over time. Although water is filling, it has no kilojoules, so it helps walkers access stored body fat sooner. You can add a squeeze of lemon or lime for extra flavour. It may seem a little strange, but you may need to drink water when you're not that thirsty. Our thirst mechanism is not that effective, and often triggers hunger instead of thirst when we are partially dehydrated. The body loses around 6 to 8 glasses of water each day, so try your best to replace it. This keeps your body well hydrated, reduces hunger pangs and boosts your metabolic rate.

 Science says – Soft drinks are the new cigarettes

Some nutrition experts now argue that soft drinks and other sugar-sweetened drinks are the primary cause of our modern obesity epidemic.

Strategy 8 – Forget the fads, celebrity diets and magic pills

No single food strategy, pill, powder or diet, including Atkins, low fat, low carb, or low kilojoule, is the answer in itself. Many popular diets succeed in the short term because they drastically restrict kilojoules, and you lose water and muscle weight. But this slows down your metabolism, and when you go off the diet, it's even harder to lose weight again in the future. What's more, you feel hungry, tired, anti-social and maybe even a little irritable. It's not a great way to live. The way you eat to lose weight has to be the way you continue to eat if you want to keep it off. So it makes sense to avoid eating plans that eliminate whole food groups, or deprive you of your favourite foods. I have seen every diet under the sun, argued with clients and doctors, and had people bail me up in shopping centres trying to justify the latest miracle diet or celebrity secret they have just discovered in a magazine. I have never seen a diet plan that works for everyone, or that pleases all the so-called experts. That's why the diet plan I have given you for the 8-week challenge is flexible. There's good nutrition and healthy, fat-burning, low kilojoule foods, but there's also variety, taste and easy-to-find foods. Now that's something that you can stick to.

Science says – Forget the quick fix

A recent study that reviewed numerous popular diet methods found that most based their evidence of success on testimonials from short-term results. It was found that fad diets don't bring about long-term weight loss, and may even be harmful to your long-term health.

Strategy 9 – Adjust your kilojoule intake for inactivity or indulgence

It's important to make adjustments to your kilojoule intake according to your activity levels. On the days you don't exercise, try to reduce your portion sizes a little, especially at night. You won't be burning off as many kilojoules that day, so try not to eat as many. And because food is often the centrepiece of socialising and celebrations, there will be times when you eat, drink and be merry. You should enjoy these times without guilt, but you can significantly reduce the impact these indulgences have on your body shape by making a few modifications. Adjust your eating throughout the day. For example, if you have had toast for breakfast and sandwiches for lunch, try to have a low-carbohydrate dinner. Alternatively, you can have a low-carbohydrate lunch when you know you are having a big dinner. You can also do a little extra exercise on the day, or do more on the day after. Try to think of one of my favourite quotes: 'If you eat it, burn it. If you drink it, earn it.'

Strategy 10 – Don't snack if you're inactive

There is a school of thought that snacking, or grazing, is helpful for weight control, as it speeds up your metabolism. By spreading your kilojoule intake over five smaller meals, instead of two or three larger ones, you will be more likely to use up kilojoules as you go instead of storing the excess. While I believe this strategy to be useful for some people, it can also be detrimental if you don't reduce the portion size of your main meals. If you snack, but continue to eat large main meals, your kilojoule intake goes up, and your metabolism would be unlikely to speed up enough to cover for it. The quality of your snacks is also an issue. A lot of the traditional snack foods available today are junk foods, or junk foods marketed as a healthy snack. Stick to fruits, vegetables, wholegrains, lean protein and low-fat yoghurt.

Fat-burning snack guidelines

- If you are active, enjoy five mini meals each day comprising breakfast, morning tea (or a second breakfast), lunch, afternoon tea and dinner
- Try to eat smaller portions at lunch and dinner
- Snack less, or don't snack at all on the days you don't exercise
- Avoid snacking before going to sleep
- Snack on healthy foods like fruit, yoghurt or a small portion of nuts
- Limit your intake of high-fat snacks
- Avoid snacking if you drink alcohol

Strategy 11 – Always eat breakfast

If you are determined to lose weight and reduce body fat, make sure you eat breakfast every day. There are several health benefits associated with eating breakfast, such as a faster metabolism, increased energy and a reduction in food cravings. It is a quick, healthy meal that requires little or no preparation. Breakfast foods such as fruit, cereal, toast or skim milk smoothies are very easy to make, and provide fibre with very little fat. If you don't feel like breakfast, it's possible the portion size of your evening meal is too large. Cut back on your dinner, and you will feel like eating breakfast. See Chapter 8 for more information on breakfast, and some tasty recipes to get you going in the morning.

Science says – The breakfast bonus

Studies have shown that a high-fibre breakfast helps to reduce the total amount of kilojoules you eat for the rest of the day.

Strategy 12 – Eat more food prepared at home

When you eat foods prepared by someone else, you are giving away control of your diet. It's hard to know exactly how the food is prepared and how many kilojoules you are consuming. It becomes an even bigger problem when there are so many indulgences available (pizza Friday, dinner out Saturday, burger Sunday), that people don't eat healthy foods the majority of the time.

Even when you try to make healthy choices, you could still end up with a kilojoule fest. For example, you could choose a tomato sauce for your pasta, but the mince could be high fat, the onions cooked in butter, and the pasta drizzled with oil. Obviously, eating food prepared by friends, restaurants, cafés and fast food outlets can still be part of a healthy-eating plan, but not regularly if you want success. When you prepare your own meals, you know exactly what ingredients have been used, and how the meal was prepared. Unless foods prepared at home are the foundation of your diet, you will find it hard to get results. If lack of time is a factor, cook while you watch television, and make sauces and soups in bulk so you can freeze the leftovers.

 Science says – The price of convenience

Convenience food, more commonly known as junk food, makes up a fifth of every dollar spent on food in Australia, which is more than double what it was 10 years ago. For every dollar spent promoting healthy food, there's about $10 spent promoting junk.

Strategy 13 – Don't beat yourself up if you indulge occasionally

Don't deprive yourself. Food is one of life's pleasures, and it's not healthy to eliminate your favourite foods or treats. You can still enjoy small portions of high=kilojoule foods once in a while. It's all right to break the rules now and then, as long as it's no more than once a week. It's how you eat most of the time that will have the biggest impact on your body shape, not what you do occasionally. I would discourage you from having a 'junk day', but a junk meal might serve a purpose when you are starting out. It helps to start a new diet plan knowing that you don't have to completely eliminate your favourite foods. It will feel a whole lot more achievable. Over time, healthy eating will become a habit, and you may not even feel like having a junk meal anymore.

 Science says – No support for junk day

There's a theory that a weekly junk day or high-fat meal can help kick-start your metabolism, preventing your body from adapting to a lower kilojoule intake. However, don't use this as a green light to binge, as there is no scientific evidence to back this up.

Strategy 14 – Eat less fat-storing foods

There are some specific foods that you really want to cut out, or cut back significantly on, if you want to achieve life-changing weight and fat loss. These foods really put the brakes on you getting results. You don't have to cut them out completely, or cut them all out at once, but over time, your body will thank you by having less of these fat cell favourites.

10 fat-storing foods to cut back on

1   Full-fat dairy products
2   Butter and margarine
3   Soft drinks
4   Fruit juice
5   Alcohol
6   Sugar
7   Low-fat products
8   White processed foods
9   Fast food
10 Fatty, processed meats

1 – Full-fat dairy products

Foods such as ice cream, cheese, sour cream, thickened cream, full-fat milk and cream cheese are all extremely high in fat and kilojoules. Because the fat is an animal fat, and therefore saturated, these foods are full of the type of fats that are most likely to balloon your fat cells. Even the reduced-fat varieties are often very high in fat, such as reduced-fat sour cream, and reduced-fat cheese. Have them in small portions, and check the food labels for the lowest-fat varieties. Skim milk, cottage cheese, low-fat ricotta, low-fat yoghurt and low-fat cream cheese are all good fat-burning foods.

2 – Butter and margarine

Butter and margarine are virtually pure dietary fat, and are loaded with fat-storing kilojoules. What's more, the type of fat in both spreads is detrimental to your heart health. One tablespoon of butter or margarine has a whopping 16 grams of fat and 610 kilojoules. If fat loss and weight control is your goal, then try to minimise your intake of these spreads. The best choice is neither. Look for healthier, lower-kilojoule alternatives to add flavour to your bread, such as low-fat cream cheese, spreadable cottage cheese, low-fat mayonnaise, chutney, relish and pickles. Use an oil spray for cooking purposes, as you tend to use less fat and kilojoules.

3 - Soft drinks

Soft drinks are loaded with sugar, yet offer no fullness or nutrients for all those kilojoules you get. One typical can of soft drink contains 10 teaspoons of sugar, and takes about 20 minutes of walking to burn off. The phosphoric acid responsible for the fizz is even bad for your bones. Soft drinks are a nutritional disaster, and I would encourage you to avoid them like a bad smell. The diet varieties are obviously much lower in kilojoules, and are a better choice if you want to lose weight and body fat. However, I worry about the long-term consequences of artificial sweeteners, and encourage you to have them only in moderation.

4 - Fruit juice

If your goal is fat loss, fruit juice is virtually no different to soft drink. It's full of kilojoules, and doesn't fill you up. People assume it's healthy because it comes from fruit. But comparing juice to fruit is like comparing white rice to brown rice. Processing removes the fibre, vitamins and minerals from the original healthy food, leaving you lots of kilojoules and little else to fill you up. I encourage you to include fruit juice in your diet only after you have lost weight and body fat, not while you are trying to lose it. If you really must have juice, water it down, or try a fruit frappé, where the whole edible part of the fruit is consumed.

5 - Alcohol

Alcohol is an enjoyable and social part of life for many, but it also helps your fat cells celebrate their existence. It's difficult, if not impossible, to lose body fat if you binge drink, or drink every day. Your body can't store alcohol, but you have to burn off the highly concentrated kilojoules in alcohol before you burn off the kilojoules you eat. What's more, you can't lose weight until you burn off not only the alcohol and food kilojoules, but also the excess kilojoules you have stored in your fat cells. If you do drink, it's important to balance out your alcohol intake with other strategies that can keep you on track. Try drinking less, spacing out your drinks with a glass of water, drinking low-alcohol or low-kilojoule beers, do extra exercise, avoid snacks while you drink and make sure you have alcohol-free days.

6 - Sugar

Sugar is high in kilojoules and low in nutrients, so try to cut back if your goal is to reduce body fat. Sugar is one of the top food additives in Australia, and is especially high in treat items such as chocolate, ice cream, cakes, biscuits and pastries. These foods are also extremely high in fat. When a food that is high in sugar also contains fat, the insulin released to store the sugar will also encourage the storage of dietary fat. Have these types of foods less often, and in smaller quantities.

7 – Low-fat products

I would forgive you for thinking that low-fat products would be listed as fat-burning foods, not fat-storing. But there is a difference between a food, and a product. Genuine low-fat foods grow in fields and trees (fruits, vegetables, wholegrains, legumes), while many low-fat, fat-free and reduced-fat products come in bright packets with numerous claims about their benefits. It might be 97 per cent fat free – but who cares? Is it also low in kilojoules and sugar, or high in fibre, protein and nutrients? Don't get roped in. You won't get great results living on low-fat varieties of cakes, biscuits, ice cream, muffins or low-fat biscuits. The reduced fat content is often replaced with sugar, and while you may be consuming less fat, there is very little difference in kilojoules. There can also be a tendency to consume larger portions of fat-reduced products, or consume additional full-fat foods afterwards because you think you have made a healthy choice. Look for low-fat products with significantly fewer kilojoules than the full-fat varieties, or have smaller portions less often.

8 – White processed foods

All grain foods raise blood sugar, which is not ideal for weight control, but some do it at a faster rate than others. The worst culprits are highly refined carbohydrate foods, such as white bread, white pasta, white rice, white flour products (biscuits, cakes, muffins) and low-fibre breakfast cereals. These high-kilojoule, low-fullness foods are absorbed quickly and used first for fuel by your body, displacing fat as an energy source and making it more available for storage. There is even a theory that your body craves larger portions of processed foods because, proportionally, they are so low in vitamins and minerals that your body needs more of them to meet its needs.

9 – Fast food

Call it junk food, fast food, convenience food, or take away, just do your best to avoid it. Foods such as pizza, hamburgers, fried chicken, hot chips and battered foods are not going to help you lose weight or get into shape. While you probably already know this, it's applying that knowledge that matters. These foods taste good, and people say that you've got to enjoy life. But an unhealthy, unwell and out-of-shape life is not exactly living life to the full. Don't use these types of foods as a reward for a big walk, or a good week. If you can't live without the junk, try to enjoy this type of food on a fortnightly to monthly basis. Just to be clear, I don't mean have pizza once a fortnight, hamburgers once a fortnight and hot chips once a fortnight. I mean have only *one* of these types of foods per fortnight total. That way, your mind knows you have not eliminated them from your diet, but they aren't the foundation of your diet (or your fat cells).

10 – Fatty, processed meats

Processed meats like sausages, ham, luncheon meat, bacon, salami, hot dogs and hamburger mince are a leading source of fat in the average diet. They are loaded with kilojoules, saturated fats, nitrates and salt, so they're not exactly your heart's best friend. The longer the shelf life of these products, the more it tends to shorten yours. Fortunately, there are healthier alternatives. Look for lean meats and mince instead of sausages, hot dogs and hamburger mince; have lean ham, shredded chicken breast or tuna instead of ham or luncheon meat; and try artichoke hearts or sun dried tomatoes instead of salami. Your heart and your waist will thank you for it.

Science says – Processed meats linked with diabetes

Researchers found that people who ate 5 or more servings a week of processed meat like hot dogs, bacon and luncheon meats suffered a 43 per cent increased risk of getting diabetes compared with those who ate less than one serving a week.

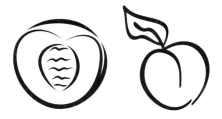

7

The Walk Off Weight
8-week challenge

'Every great journey starts with a few small steps.'

How to use this chapter to lose weight

If you really want something (weight and fat loss), why not challenge yourself to achieve it? Why not try something different to help get the results you really want? Deep down inside, you know that walking and healthy eating works. I know it works too – I've seen it work for literally thousands of my personal training clients and Gutbusters guys. I want it to work for you too, so I've mapped out a plan to change your life in 56 days. In this chapter you will find an 8-week, day-by-day guide to walking for 3 different levels and stages of fitness. There's also space for you to plan out your new eating plan based on the strategies in Chapter 6 and the recipes and fast feast ideas that we'll cover in Chapter 8. If you challenge yourself and commit to the 8 weeks, you will lose weight, burn fat, get fitter and change your body shape. To help guide you through, there are 3 easy steps to carry out to help you get the most out of the 8-week challenge. The three steps are:

- **Step 1** Test your readiness to start a walking program
- **Step 2** Determine what level you should start at
- **Step 3** Start walking, and fill out daily worksheets

Step 1 – Test your readiness to start a walking program

Is your health at risk?

You are about to begin a new exercise program for health, fitness, fat loss and a new quality of life. What's more, you have chosen the best form of exercise to start with – walking. Walking is one of the most gradual and sensible activities when starting a new exercise program. It's pretty exciting stuff, and I'm sure you can't wait to start, but even so, I encourage you to read Chapter 12. Here you will learn more about stretching and injury prevention, the importance of warming up, cooling down, staying supple, and avoiding the common problems walkers face. There may also be some circumstances in which you need a medical clearance to begin an exercise program. Consult your doctor if any of these conditions apply to you:

- pregnancy
- diabetes
- chest pain, especially during exertion
- family history of heart disease
- asthma, arthritis, epilepsy or obesity
- high blood pressure
- inactivity for 12 months or more
- previous heart attack or stroke
- aged 55 years or older

Assess yourself before you start

It's a good idea to record a few basic health and fitness measures before you start a new exercise program. This gives you a benchmark against which you can measure your progress down the track. It can also be a motivational boost to have a time or measurement that you can improve upon. Why not fill out the details in the table following, and check out your improvement after the 8-week challenge. You don't have to use them all, and you might have your own measure, like how a particular pair of jeans fits, but try to find a measurement that means something to you.

Measurement	Today	8 weeks	12 months
	__ / __ / __	__ / __ / __	__ / __ / __
Body weight (Make sure this is not your only measure)			
Body fat percentage (From special scales, or from a professional assessment)			
Waist in centimetres/inches (Measure at the narrowest point)			
Buttocks in centimetres/inches (Measure at the widest point)			
2 kilometre walk in minutes * (Map out a 2 km walk with your car odometer. You can also test your pulse rate at the end of the walk.)			

Resting pulse per minute (Take from the thumb side of your wrist first thing in the morning. Count the pulse for 20 seconds and multiply by 3.)			
General wellbeing (Give yourself a score out of 10 on how you feel about your energy levels and overall wellness.)			

If you are very unfit or very overweight, take this nice and easy.

Step 2 – Determine what level you should start at

You will notice the daily worksheets have three different levels for walkers – the beginner program, the Walk Off Weight program, and the advanced program. To help you decide which level is best for you, see which description best suits you.

The beginner program

The beginner program is suitable if any or all of these are relevant to you.
- You can only walk at a leisurely pace for 5 to 10 minutes comfortably.
- You are very overweight.
- You haven't exercised for at least 12 months.
- You have a heart condition (and clearance from your doctor).

You will still lose some weight and fat on this program, but it's more focused on getting some movement back into your life. You can accumulate your walking minutes over the day instead of doing them all at once at this stage. The beginner program will prepare you for the Walk Off Weight program.

The Walk Off Weight program

The Walk Off Weight program is suitable if any or all of these are relevant to you.
- You can walk at a moderate pace for 20 to 30 minutes comfortably.
- You are overweight, but not extremely overweight.
- You haven't exercised for a while.

Your walks have a variety of different durations and intensities. If you feel like doing a light walk after your more intense walks, feel free. My hope is that by the end of the 8 weeks, you will have lost some weight, and feel ready for the advanced program.

The advanced program

The advanced program is suitable if any or all of these are relevant to you.
- You have been active with other vigorous activities.
- You can walk at a fast pace for 30 to 40 minutes comfortably.
- You already walk occasionally, but you want to take your walking to a new level.

Before starting the advanced program, please make sure you read Chapter 9. You will get a better understanding of the cross-training and interval-training strategies I have incorporated into your program.

What if I have chosen the wrong level?

The durations and intensities I have set are only a guide. You may find after a few days that the duration, and/or intensity of your walks are too easy, and you want to work above those set out in the activity journal. Either take yourself up to the next level, or continue to work above the planned guidelines. You can even go up a level just for a day or two throughout the 8 weeks for a bit of variety. Feel free to upgrade yourself to the next level at any stage. If you are finding the program too hard, just drop back your intensity or duration or both, and work through the 8 weeks at your own pace. You can also drop down to an easier program level at any time. This is a challenge, not a competition, so give your body time to adjust, and enjoy.

Step 3 – Start walking, and fill out the daily worksheets

Planning your walks and meals, and then writing down the details of what you actually did (how hard and how long you walked for) and what you actually ate (above and beyond what you planned to eat) is a real key to success in weight and fat loss. You don't need to write things down forever, but it can really help to smooth out the bumps when you start a new program of exercise and change the way you eat. Keeping a written record for 8 weeks is a genuine commitment to change and to getting results. It should only take you a few minutes each day. Each of the 56 daily worksheets includes:
- a motivational quote
- an activity plan, with guidelines on walking for duration and exertion at three different levels
- an activity journal, with blank spaces for you to fill in the details of your actual workouts
- a meal planner for you to detail what you intend to eat that day
- a food diary, where you can fill in what you actually ate that day
- trainer's notes to keep you well informed and on track

Filling in the activity journal

I've set some exercise goals for you in the 'planned activity' section of each daily worksheet. Now it's time to get out there and get moving. It's time to fill in the 'activity journal', and record the actual details of your walks. The walking levels I refer to in the 'planned activity' section are based on the rate of perceived exertion scale covered in Chapter 3. It might seem easier just to record how long you walked for, but don't forget that walking too slowly is one of the main reasons why most walkers don't get great results. I encourage you to bookmark the rate of perceived exertion scale (RPE) scale on page 12, and refer to it every day. It's an easy way to measure the intensity of your walks. If you have a heart rate monitor, pedometer, or GPS device that measures your average speed, you may wish to enter data from those devices as well. Why not make Day 1 today?

Sample activity journal

	Planned activity	Activity journal
Beginner	Walk at level 2 (very easy) for 5 to 10 minutes	12 minutes at level 2
Walk off weight	Walk at level 3 (somewhat easy) for 25 minutes	
Advanced	Walk at level 5 (somewhat hard) for 30 minutes	

What about rest days and missed days?

If you are a beginner, don't bother scanning through the 8-week challenge to see where the rest days are. There aren't any. But I'm pretty sure you'll schedule your own. It's more than likely you will miss a day or two throughout the 8-week challenge. So let me stress that you should not worry, and that you should just get right back into it. Jump straight back on the horse, and don't use it as an excuse to give up. If your body is sore and you feel exhausted, have a break, but try to make up the time on a different day. I have also scheduled some light walks every week to help your body recover. Try to get into the habit of walking every day. The same goes for the Walk Off Weight program. If you want to lose weight and get results, give your fat cells the message every day that they are not wanted. Challenge yourself to still be walking in 8 weeks' time. There's no doubt it will improve your health and help you lose weight. There's no better time to start than now. Advanced walkers are training at a higher intensity, so I have scheduled a choice between a rest day, or a very light day every week. Add your own light activities, or combine the activities I have suggested.

Filling in the menu planner

Planning your meals in advance is a proven way to improve your diet and lose weight. You'll be less likely to buy junk food, and it makes initial changes to your diet easier. When planning your meals, consider using the recipes in Chapter 8. I have included 7 recipes each for breakfast, lunch, dinner and snacks – that's one for each day of the week. Most of the recipes have variations for you to try, and you will also find several fast feast ideas to tempt your taste buds. You can incorporate other recipes, but try to stick with healthy low-kilojoule foods, and keep your portion sizes under control. Try to plan out 4 to 7 days at a time, and then use your meal planner to make out your shopping list.

Sample meal planner

	Menu planner	Food diary
Breakfast	Soft Swiss Muesli (see page 114)	
Lunch	Tuna salad (see page 119)	
Dinner	Chilli con carne (see page 127)	
Snacks	1 x 200 gram yoghurt mid-morning 1 pear mid-afternoon	
Glasses of water		☐☐☐☐☐☐☐☐

Filling in the food diary

Your food diary is where you record what you actually did eat, as opposed to what you planned to eat. Even with the best of intentions, everyone will stray from the path at some point. Your food diary allows you to keep track of your diet, your binges, times when you are most likely to stray, and patterns in your eating habits. If you do eat what is written down in the menu planner, just leave the food diary blank for that relevant meal, or place a tick. If you eat something that you hadn't planned, write it down. You can also use the space to make comments about how you felt, or why you changed your plan. There is also a place down the bottom to tick off your 8 glasses of water throughout the day.

Sample food diary

	Menu planner	Food diary
Breakfast	Soft Swiss Muesli (see page 114)	☑
Lunch	Tuna Salad (see page 119)	☑
Dinner	Chilli Con Carne (see page 127)	Pasta with tomato sauce and 1 glass of wine (Asked out to dinner at last minute)
Snacks	1 x 200 gram yoghurt mid-morning 1 pear mid-afternoon	☑ 1 x apple
Glasses of water		☑☑☑☑☑☑☑☑

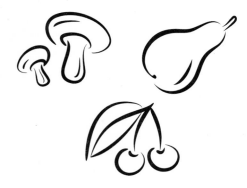

Day 1

Motivational quote of the day

'The act of taking the first step is what separates the winners from the losers.' – Brian Tracy, *motivational speaker.*

	Planned activity	Activity journal
Beginner	Walk at level 2 (very easy) for 10 minutes	
Walk Off Weight	Walk at level 3 (somewhat easy) for 35 minutes	
Advanced	Walk at level 5 (somewhat hard) for 35 minutes	

	Menu planner	Food diary
Breakfast		
Lunch		
Dinner		
Snacks		
Glasses of water		☐ ☐ ☐ ☐ ☐ ☐ ☐

Trainer's notes – Taking that first step

Today is the start of your 8-week challenge. The time for reading and contemplation is over. It's great that you are taking this opportunity to lose weight, improve your health and maximise your energy levels. This is the day you will kick-start your walking program into gear, and generate some forward momentum. If you are a beginner, take things really easy today. If you feel any pain or discomfort, slow down your speed, or even take a rest.

Day 2

Motivational quote of the day

'The only thing that will stop you from fulfilling your dreams is you.'
— Tom Bradley

	Planned activity	Activity journal
Beginner	Walk at level 2 (very easy) for 10 minutes	
Walk Off Weight	Walk at level 4 (moderate) for 25 minutes	
Advanced	Strength training for 20 minutes Walk at level 6 (hard) for 10 minutes	

	Menu planner	Food diary
Breakfast		
Lunch		
Dinner		
Snacks		
Glasses of water		☐☐☐☐☐☐☐☐

Trainer's notes – Find a motivating force

Try to have a clear understanding of why you want to lose body fat, as it can be a powerful and personal motivating force that kicks you into action. What are the reasons you want to lose body fat, and what will happen if you don't do something about it? Write down your thoughts and feelings, or at least contemplate your answers.

Day 3

Motivational quote of the day

'The secret of getting ahead is getting started. The secret of getting started is breaking your complex, overwhelming tasks into small manageable tasks, and then starting on the first one.' – Mark Twain

	Planned activity	Activity journal
Beginner	Walk at level 2 (very easy) for 10 minutes	
Walk Off Weight	Walk at level 3 (somewhat easy) for 35 minutes	
Advanced	Walk at level 4 (moderate) for 45 to 60 minutes	

	Menu planner	Food diary
Breakfast		
Lunch		
Dinner		
Snacks		
Glasses of water		☐☐☐☐☐☐☐☐

Trainer's notes – Don't give up now

Most people who start a new diet give up after 3 days. The drop-out rate is so high because people try unbalanced diets that are so far removed from how people can eat, or want to eat. People who finally decide to take action want dramatic results, so they try drastic changes hoping to meet their unrealistic expectations. That's why I encourage you to take things easy at the start, and feel encouraged to continue.

Day 4

Motivational quote of the day

'All things are difficult before they are easy.' – Thomas Fuller

	Planned activity	Activity journal
Beginner	Walk at level 2 (very easy) for 10 minutes	
Walk Off Weight	Walk at level 4 (moderate) for 25 minutes	
Advanced	Cross training (cycling, paddling, sports, running) for 40 to 60 minutes	

	Menu planner	Food diary
Breakfast		
Lunch		
Dinner		
Snacks		
Glasses of water		☐☐☐☐☐☐☐☐

Trainer's notes – Welcome change

If you don't change your eating habits or activity levels, you won't change your body shape. So why not embrace change – welcome it. The best changes to make are gradual, and built up over time. Don't try to change it all in 1 day, or even 1 week. Stick with me for the 8 weeks, I promise you it's worth it.

Day 5

Motivational quote of the day

'The difference between the impossible and the possible lies in a person's determination.' – Tommy Lasorda

	Planned activity	Activity journal
Beginner	Walk at level 2 (very easy) for 10 minutes	
Walk Off Weight	Walk at level 3 (somewhat easy) for 35 minutes	
Advanced	Interval training Level 7 (very hard) walk/run for 30 to 60 seconds x 15 Level 4 (moderate) walk for 60 to 90 seconds x 15	

	Menu planner	Food diary
Breakfast		
Lunch		
Dinner		
Snacks		
Glasses of water		☐☐☐☐☐☐☐☐

Trainer's notes – Friday on my mind

Studies have shown that as the week wears on, people lose their drive to eat well and exercise. It doesn't necessarily mean they drop out, but they are more health conscious from Monday to Thursday, and then fall away on Friday, Saturday and Sunday. Be aware of this pattern, and do all you can to see out the full week.

Day 6

Motivational quote of the day

'We should be taught not to wait for inspiration to start a thing. Action always generates inspiration. Inspiration seldom generates action.' – Frank Tibolt

	Planned activity	Activity journal
Beginner	Walk at level 2 (very easy) for 10 minutes	
Walk Off Weight	Walk at level 4 (moderate) for 25 minutes Walk at level 2 (very easy) for 15 minutes	
Advanced	Strength training for 20 minutes Walk at level 6 (hard) for 10 minutes	

	Menu planner	Food diary
Breakfast		
Lunch		
Dinner		
Snacks		
Glasses of water		☐☐☐☐☐☐☐☐

Trainer's notes – Don't be lazy after your walk

Studies have shown that people who do intense exercise, and then do nothing for the rest of the day, can burn off less total kilojoules than people who don't exercise, but perform incidental movement throughout the day. Be active in as many ways as you can. Don't be lazy or stop moving about just because you have checked exercise off your daily list.

Day 7

Motivational quote of the day

'There's a very positive relationship between people's ability to accomplish any task and the time they're willing to spend on it.'
– Joyce Brothers

	Planned activity	Activity journal
Beginner	Walk at level 2 (very easy) for 10 to 15 minutes	
Walk Off Weight	Walk at level 2 (very easy) for 50 minutes	
Advanced	Rest day Level 3 (somewhat easy) walk for 30 to 60 minutes, or do a session of stretching	

	Menu planner	Food diary
Breakfast		
Lunch		
Dinner		
Snacks		
Glasses of water		☐☐☐☐☐☐☐☐

Trainer's notes – Well done – that's Week 1

You have made a start, and hopefully, stuck to the program. What might have seemed difficult a week ago now seems achievable. You can look forward to next week with more confidence and self-belief. Focus on the small successes, and try to learn from any setbacks.

Day 8

Motivational quote of the day

'Success seems to be connected with action. Successful people keep moving. They make mistakes, but they don't quit.' – Conrad Hilton

	Planned activity	Activity journal
Beginner	Walk at level 2 (very easy) for 15 minutes	
Walk Off Weight	Walk at level 3 (somewhat easy) for 35 minutes	
Advanced	Walk at level 5 (somewhat hard) for 40 minutes	

	Menu planner	Food diary
Breakfast		
Lunch		
Dinner		
Snacks		
Glasses of water		☐☐☐☐☐☐☐

Trainer's notes – Excuses are fattening

There's always an excuse for why overweight people can't exercise, can't push themselves hard today, can't change their diet yet, can't drink less alcohol this weekend, can't find the time, can't get out of bed early this week, and don't feel motivated. But it's these very excuses that are keeping them from losing body fat. For every excuse, there is an alternative or solution, another way to make the sort of choices that will improve your health and make a difference. If you want results, find a way to get out of the excuse-making mindset.

Day 9

Motivational quote of the day

'People are always blaming their circumstances for what they are. I don't believe in circumstances. The people who get on in this world are the people who get up and look for the circumstances they want, and if they can't find them, make them.' – George Bernard Shaw

	Planned activity	Activity journal
Beginner	Walk at level 2 (very easy) for 15 minutes	
Walk Off Weight	Walk at level 4 (moderate) for 25 minutes	
Advanced	Strength training for 25 minutes Walk at level 6 (hard) for 10 minutes	

	Menu planner	Food diary
Breakfast		
Lunch		
Dinner		
Snacks		
Glasses of water		☐☐☐☐☐☐☐☐

Trainer's notes – Fighting those food cravings

Changing your diet often leads to strong cravings for foods that almost certainly won't help you achieve your goals. Some strategies to help you overcome food cravings include identifying and preventing situations or emotions that trigger cravings, drinking plenty of water, eating smaller amounts more often and meeting your desire with a little of what you fancy. Small portions allow you to satisfy your taste buds and meet your anticipation without the feeling of total deprivation.

Day 10

Motivational quote of the day

'Action may not always be happiness, but there is no happiness without action.' – Benjamin Disraeli

	Planned activity	Activity journal
Beginner	Walk at level 2 (very easy) for 15 minutes	
Walk Off Weight	Walk at level 3 (somewhat easy) for 35 minutes	
Advanced	Walk at level 4 (moderate) for 45 to 60 minutes	

	Menu planner	Food diary
Breakfast		
Lunch		
Dinner		
Snacks		
Glasses of water		☐☐☐☐☐☐☐☐

Trainer's notes – Don't eat more after walking

Exercise may temporarily lower your appetite immediately after a good walk, but within a few hours, you may get hungry. This is especially true in women, who have a stronger hunger response from exercise than men. This is the body's natural defence mechanism to protect your existing fat stores. Drink plenty of water, and keep your portion sizes under control so you don't blow all your good work.

Day 11

Motivational quote of the day

'All great achievements require time.' – Maya Angelou

	Planned activity	Activity journal
Beginner	Walk at level 2 (very easy) for 15 minutes	
Walk Off Weight	Walk at level 4 (moderate) for 25 minutes	
Advanced	Cross training (cycling, paddling, sports, running) for 40 to 60 minutes	

	Menu planner	Food diary
Breakfast		
Lunch		
Dinner		
Snacks		
Glasses of water		☐☐☐☐☐☐☐☐

Trainer's notes – Make the necessary adjustments

Remember that the founding principle of fat loss is to use more kilojoules through exercise than you consume (food). When you look at this from a daily perspective, if you have an inactive day, you won't need as many kilojoules to fuel your body. Try to eat a little less on the days you don't exercise to maximise fat loss.

Day 12

Motivational quote of the day

'Success is the ability to go from one failure to another with no loss of enthusiasm.' – Winston Churchill

	Planned activity	Activity journal
Beginner	Walk at level 2 (very easy) for 15 minutes	
Walk Off Weight	Walk at level 3 (somewhat easy) for 35 minutes	
Advanced	Interval training. Find as many hills as you can during your walk, and walk as fast as you can up each one	

	Menu planner	Food diary
Breakfast		
Lunch		
Dinner		
Snacks		
Glasses of water		☐☐☐☐☐☐☐☐

Trainer's notes – The weekend warrior

Most people have more time on the weekends. If you only manage to fit in a few walks during the weekdays, do two big long walks on both Saturday and Sunday. It's also a good time to plan out your food for the week, and even prepare a few meals in advance. It's better to be a weekend warrior than a couch potato.

Day 13

Motivational quote of the day

'Great things are done by a series of small things brought together.'
— Vincent Van Gogh

	Planned activity	Activity journal
Beginner	Walk at level 2 (very easy) for 15 minutes	
Walk Off Weight	Walk at level 4 (moderate) for 25 minutes Walk at level 2 (very easy) for 15 minutes	
Advanced	Strength training for 25 minutes Walk at level 6 (hard) for 10 minutes	

	Menu planner	Food diary
Breakfast		
Lunch		
Dinner		
Snacks		
Glasses of water		☐☐☐☐☐☐☐☐

Trainer's notes – It's all in the planning

Preparation is an often forgotten factor in determining your success at achieving health and fitness goals. Think about what actions you need to take to get results. It might be to plan your meals in advance, to get your workout clothes ready before you go to bed, or to take fruit with you so you have a healthy option when you're out and about.

Day 14

Motivational quote of the day

'Whoever wants to reach a distant goal must take many small steps.'
— *Helmut Schmidt*

	Planned activity	Activity journal
Beginner	Walk at level 2 (very easy) for 15 to 20 minutes	
Walk Off Weight	Walk at level 5 (somewhat hard) for 20 minutes	
Advanced	Rest day Level 3 (somewhat easy) walk for 30 to 60 minutes, or do a yoga class/video	

	Menu planner	Food diary
Breakfast		
Lunch		
Dinner		
Snacks		
Glasses of water		☐☐☐☐☐☐☐☐

Trainer's notes – Congratulations – you've completed Week 2

Well done. If you are a beginner, you should be starting to breathe a little easier during your walks. If you are walking off weight, you are on the right course. Keep working on your diet, and make sure to keep your portions down. If you are an advanced walker, you should be starting to push yourself to a new level. Keep it up, and let's finish what we've started.

Day 15

Motivational quote of the day

'If we have our own "why" of life, we can clear almost any "how".'
— Friedrich Nietzsche

	Planned activity	Activity journal
Beginner	Walk at level 2 (very easy) for 20 minutes	
Walk Off Weight	Walk at level 3 (somewhat easy) for 40 minutes	
Advanced	Walk at level 5 (somewhat hard) for 45 minutes	

	Menu planner	Food diary
Breakfast		
Lunch		
Dinner		
Snacks		
Glasses of water		☐☐☐☐☐☐☐☐

Trainer's notes – Walk instead of wasting time

Nothing great has ever come from watching television. Time that you spend playing computer games, surfing the internet or watching DVDs can really be put to better use. Instead of winding down in front of the idiot box at the end of the day, why not go for a walk? Not only can it help you de-stress and clear your mind, but you can burn off some of your dinner as well.

Day 16

Motivational quote of the day

'Even if you're on the right track, you'll get run over if you just sit there.' – *Will Rogers*

	Planned activity	Activity journal
Beginner	Walk at level 2 (very easy) for 20 minutes	
Walk Off Weight	Walk at level 4 (moderate) or 30 minutes	
Advanced	Strength training for 25 minutes Walk at level 6 (hard) for 15 minutes	

	Menu planner	Food diary
Breakfast		
Lunch		
Dinner		
Snacks		
Glasses of water		☐☐☐☐☐☐☐☐

Trainer's notes – Make your bad choices better

Healthy eating means making good food choices most of the time, and unhealthy choices less often. Another consideration is to make better choices when you make bad ones. If you have a craving for French fries, choose the small size. Have 1 glass of wine instead of 2. Buy an individually wrapped chocolate instead of a whole block. You can still enjoy your foods, and minimise the impact on your healthy-eating plan.

Day 17

Motivational quote of the day

'It is not the strongest of the species that survive, nor the most intelligent, but the one most responsive to change.' – Charles Darwin

	Planned activity	Activity journal
Beginner	Walk at level 2 (very easy) for 20 minutes	
Walk Off Weight	Walk at level 3 (somewhat easy) for 40 minutes	
Advanced	Walk at level 4 (moderate) for 45 to 60 minutes	

	Menu planner	Food diary
Breakfast		
Lunch		
Dinner		
Snacks		
Glasses of water		☐☐☐☐☐☐☐☐

Trainer's notes – Seek out support

Let your family and friends know that you have a new health and fitness goal. Try to enlist the support of your partner or work colleagues to encourage you and be part of your journey. It's much easier if you have someone to share your thoughts and frustrations with, who can offer a little bit of motivation when you really need it.

Day 18

Motivational quote of the day

'If you really want something, and really work hard, and take advantage of opportunities, and never give up, you will find a way.'
— Jane Goodall

	Planned activity	Activity journal
Beginner	Walk at level 2 (very easy) for 20 minutes	
Walk Off Weight	Walk at level 4 (moderate) for 30 minutes	
Advanced	Cross training (cycling, paddling, sports, running) for 40 to 60 minutes	

	Menu planner	Food diary
Breakfast		
Lunch		
Dinner		
Snacks		
Glasses of water		☐ ☐ ☐ ☐ ☐ ☐ ☐ ☐

Trainer's notes – Walk – and don't delay

Try not to think too long and hard about your exercise. Just do it. People who deliberate or tell themselves they may not feel like doing exercise are less likely to actually perform exercise. Just start, even if you tell yourself you will only walk for 5 to 10 minutes. Once you actually start, you have crossed the biggest hurdle, and you might even feel like continuing for longer.

Day 19

Motivational quote of the day

'You miss 100% of the shots you never take.' – *Wayne Gretzky*

	Planned activity	Activity journal
Beginner	Walk at level 2 (very easy) for 20 minutes	
Walk Off Weight	Walk at level 3 (somewhat easy) for 40 minutes	
Advanced	Walk at level 7 (very hard) for the distance between 2 telegraph poles, and level 4 (moderate) for the next 2 poles. Try to do 20 intervals, and finish with level 5 (somewhat hard) for 20 minutes	

	Menu planner	Food diary
Breakfast		
Lunch		
Dinner		
Snacks		
Glasses of water		☐☐☐☐☐☐☐☐

Trainer's notes – Don't be embarrassed

Embarrassment has been identified as a major factor that keeps people from exercising. Unfortunately, some people get shy exercising in public. But don't worry about what other people think. Take confidence from your own actions to improve your weight and your health.

Day 20

Motivational quote of the day

'One's best success comes after his greatest disappointments.'

— Henry Ward Beecher

	Planned activity	Activity journal
Beginner	Walk at level 2 (very easy) for 20 minutes	
Walk Off Weight	Walk at level 4 (moderate) for 30 minutes Walk at level 3 (somewhat easy) for 15 minutes	
Advanced	Strength training for 25 minutes Walk at level 6 (hard) for 15 minutes	

	Menu planner	Food diary
Breakfast		
Lunch		
Dinner		
Snacks		
Glasses of water		☐☐☐☐☐☐☐☐

Trainer's notes – Meal replacements may work

Research has shown that meal replacements can be successful in helping people maintain weight loss for more than five years. Advances in food technology, improved ingredients and better taste have meant the shakes, soups, bars and prepared meals you now see in the pharmacy or supermarket may actually help, as long as you're prepared to stick with them. I suggest you don't use them every day, but use them occasionally as a fall back. They're much better than take away.

Day 21

Motivational quote of the day

'I know the price of success: dedication, hard work and an unremitting devotion to the things you want to see happen.'

– Frank Lloyd Wright

	Planned activity	Activity journal
Beginner	Walk at level 3 (somewhat easy) for 15 minutes	
Walk Off Weight	Walk at level 2 (very easy) for 55 minutes	
Advanced	Rest day Level 3 (somewhat easy) walk for 30 to 60 minutes, or do a Tai Chi class/video	

	Menu planner	Food diary
Breakfast		
Lunch		
Dinner		
Snacks		
Glasses of water		☐☐☐☐☐☐☐☐

Trainer's notes – Three weeks, and new habits are forming

It's now been 21 days since you started your new walking program, which is exactly how long it's thought to take to form a new habit. When your new behaviour becomes a habit, things become automatic instead of forced. You should start to find that you look forward to your walks, and that it's easier to fit them into your day.

Day 22

Motivational quote of the day

*'The elevator to success is out of order. You'll have to use the stairs
...one step at a time.'* – Joe Girard

	Planned activity	Activity journal
Beginner	Walk at level 2 (very easy) for 25 minutes	
Walk Off Weight	Walk at level 3 (somewhat easy) for 40 minutes	
Advanced	Walk at level 5 (somewhat hard) for 50 minutes	

	Menu planner	Food diary
Breakfast		
Lunch		
Dinner		
Snacks		
Glasses of water		☐☐☐☐☐☐☐☐

Trainer's notes – When to do weights

If your goal is to reduce body fat, lifting weights can make a difference, but so can the order of your activities. If you intend to walk and lift weights on the same day, try to do your weights first. The short bursts of intense effort during strength training will use up blood glucose, making it more likely you will burn off fat as fuel during your walk. Just make sure not to eat or drink anything but water after your weights workout to maximise the effect.

Day 23

Motivational quote of the day

'Look at a day when you are supremely satisfied at the end. It's not a day when you lounge around doing nothing; it's when you've had everything to do, and you've done it.' – Margaret Thatcher

	Planned activity	Activity journal
Beginner	Walk at level 3 (somewhat easy) for 15 minutes	
Walk Off Weight	Walk at level 4 (moderate) for 30 minutes	
Advanced	Strength training for 30 minutes Walk at level 6 (hard) for 15 minutes	

	Menu planner	Food diary
Breakfast		
Lunch		
Dinner		
Snacks		
Glasses of water		☐☐☐☐☐☐☐☐

Trainer's notes – Help to inspire others

See if you can help someone else to lose weight and improve his or her health. The best way to learn is to teach. Encouraging a friend, relative or partner to make changes is also a great way to reinforce the changes you have already made. This can give you strength in numbers and the support of someone who shares a common goal. It can also add to the enjoyment of your new healthier lifestyle.

Day 24

Motivational quote of the day

'The path to success is to take massive, determined action.'
— Anthony Robbins

	Planned activity	Activity journal
Beginner	Walk at level 2 (very easy) for 25 minutes	
Walk Off Weight	Walk at level 3 (somewhat easy) for 40 minutes	
Advanced	Walk at level 4 (moderate) for 45 to 60 minutes	

	Menu planner	Food diary
Breakfast		
Lunch		
Dinner		
Snacks		
Glasses of water		☐☐☐☐☐☐☐☐

Trainer's notes – Change your movement mindset

With a never-ending supply of labour-saving devices and gadgets, we are suffering from motion deprivation. People seek out the closest car park so they don't have to walk far, and can eat cake while someone else washes their car. But to lose body fat, you need to move more. Try to look upon extra bits of movement as an opportunity, not an inconvenience. While planned, intentional walking is vital for weight control, incidental walking can still make a difference.

Day 25

Motivational quote of the day

'When life's problems seem overwhelming, look around and see what other people are coping with. You may consider yourself fortunate.'
— Ann Landers

	Planned activity	Activity journal
Beginner	Walk at level 3 (somewhat easy) for 15 minutes	
Walk Off Weight	Walk at level 4 (moderate) for 30 minutes	
Advanced	Cross training (cycling, paddling, sports, running) for 40 to 60 minutes	

	Menu planner	Food diary
Breakfast		
Lunch		
Dinner		
Snacks		
Glasses of water		☐☐☐☐☐☐☐☐

Trainer's notes – Get out in the garden

Gardening provides a wide variety of movements that work your muscles and burn kilojoules. If you combine vigorous active movements over a long duration, such as digging, raking, pulling, walking and squatting, you can get a good whole-body workout. The more muscles involved in your activity, the more kilojoules you'll burn. Perform all movements at an energetic pace for maximum results.

Day 26

Motivational quote of the day

'Difficulties are meant to rouse, not discourage. The human spirit is to grow strong by conflict.' – *William Ellery Channing*

	Planned activity	Activity journal
Beginner	Walk at level 2 (very easy) for 25 minutes	
Walk Off Weight	Walk at level 3 (somewhat easy) for 40 minutes	
Advanced	Find the biggest flight of stairs near you, and walk as fast as you can, 1 step at a time Repeat for 20 minutes, then finish with level 5 (somewhat hard) for 20 minutes	

	Menu planner	Food diary
Breakfast		
Lunch		
Dinner		
Snacks		
Glasses of water		☐☐☐☐☐☐☐☐

Trainer's notes – Focus on the quality of your carbohydrates

When it comes to carbohydrates, it's the type you eat that makes a difference to your body fat levels, new research shows. People who are overweight do not appear to eat more carbohydrates overall than people who weigh less, but overweight people tend to eat more refined carbohydrates, such as white bread and pasta. Refined carbohydrates are also found in processed foods that contain lots of sugar.

Day 27

Motivational quote of the day

'The ability to discipline yourself to delay gratification in the short term in order to enjoy greater rewards in the long term is the indispensable prerequisite for success.' – Brian Tracy

	Planned activity	Activity journal
Beginner	Walk at level 3 (somewhat easy) for 15 minutes	
Walk Off Weight	Walk at level 4 (moderate) for 30 minutes Walk at level 3 (somewhat easy) for 15 minutes	
Advanced	Strength training for 30 minutes Walk at level 6 (hard) for 15 minutes	

	Menu planner	Food diary
Breakfast		
Lunch		
Dinner		
Snacks		
Glasses of water		☐☐☐☐☐☐☐☐

Trainer's notes – Sweet tooth or fat tooth

A recent study found that people who claim to have a sweet tooth eat 12 to 14 grams more fat a day than people who avoid sweets. This is because foods thought of as sweet treats (such as chocolate) are usually high in fat. To satisfy your sweet tooth, try fruit, or foods such as jelly babies, boiled lollies, killer pythons, marshmallows and meringue. These foods are sweet but have virtually no fat.

Day 28

Motivational quote of the day

'Winners must learn to relish change with the same enthusiasm and energy that we have resisted it in the past.' – Tom Peters

	Planned activity	Activity journal
Beginner	Walk at level 2 (very easy) for 30 minutes	
Walk Off Weight	Walk at level 2 (very easy) for 60 minutes	
Advanced	Rest day Level 3 (somewhat easy) walk for 30 to 60 minutes, or do a Pilates class/video	

	Menu planner	Food diary
Breakfast		
Lunch		
Dinner		
Snacks		
Glasses of water		☐☐☐☐☐☐☐☐

Trainer's notes – Week 4 – you are halfway there

Well done. You have completed your first month. As you look ahead at the next 4 weeks, feel confident knowing you have already achieved a month of exercise. It's also a good time to evaluate your progress. If you haven't noticed any changes, take a closer look at your diet, or increase the speed, frequency or duration of your walks.

Day 29

Motivational quote of the day

'He who would learn to fly one day must first learn to stand and walk and run and climb and dance; one cannot fly into flying.'

— Friedrich Nietzsche

	Planned activity	Activity journal
Beginner	Walk at level 3 (somewhat easy) for 20 minutes	
Walk Off Weight	Walk at level 3 (somewhat easy) for 45 minutes	
Advanced	Walk at level 6 (hard) for 35 minutes	

	Menu planner	Food diary
Breakfast		
Lunch		
Dinner		
Snacks		
Glasses of water		☐ ☐ ☐ ☐ ☐ ☐ ☐ ☐

Trainer's notes – Eat a wide variety of food

People who eat a variety of foods have been shown to be healthier than those who have a more limited diet. Eating at least 30 different types of food each day, and 40 different types of food each week, exposes your body to a wide variety of vitamins, minerals and nutrients from your diet. It's also thought to keep your metabolism functioning at it's best. Try different herbs, spices, grains, fruits and vegetables to add new colours, flavours, aroma's and textures to your diet.

Day 30

Motivational quote of the day

'The state of your life is nothing more than a reflection of your state of mind.' – Dr. Wayne W. Dyer

	Planned activity	Activity journal
Beginner	Walk at level 2 (very easy) for 30 minutes	
Walk Off Weight	Walk at level 4 (moderate) for 35 minutes	
Advanced	Strength training for 30 minutes Walk at level 6 (hard) for 20 minutes	

	Menu planner	Food diary
Breakfast		
Lunch		
Dinner		
Snacks		
Glasses of water		☐☐☐☐☐☐☐☐

Trainer's notes – Be careful when eating with friends

A recent study discovered that women who dine in the presence of others almost double the amount of food they eat compared to when they eat alone. Study participants eating in groups of friends also ate more than those in groups of strangers. It seems that socialising has a significant effect on the duration of time and the amount of kilojoules consumed during a meal.

Day 31

Motivational quote of the day

'Victory belongs to the most persevering.' – Napoleon Bonaparte

	Planned activity	Activity journal
Beginner	Walk at level 3 (somewhat easy) for 20 minutes	
Walk Off Weight	Walk at level 5 (somewhat hard) for 25 minutes	
Advanced	Walk at level 5 (somewhat hard) for 45 to 60 minutes	

	Menu planner	Food diary
Breakfast		
Lunch		
Dinner		
Snacks		
Glasses of water		☐☐☐☐☐☐☐☐

Trainer's notes – Dare to share

When you are craving a food, the most pleasure is gained from the first mouthful. So use this knowledge when you indulge, and try to share your entrées or desserts. This can help to reduce your portion size, and cut back on your kilojoule intake, reducing the impact eating out has on your health and body shape.

Day 32

Motivational quote of the day

'For every difficulty that supposedly stops a person from succeeding there are thousands who have had it a lot worse and have succeeded anyway. So can you.' – Brian Tracy

	Planned activity	Activity journal
Beginner	Walk at level 2 (very easy) for 30 minutes	
Walk Off Weight	Walk at level 3 (somewhat easy) for 45 minutes	
Advanced	Cross training (cycling, paddling, sports, running) for 40 to 60 minutes	

	Menu planner	Food diary
Breakfast		
Lunch		
Dinner		
Snacks		
Glasses of water		☐☐☐☐☐☐☐☐

Trainer's notes – Eat plenty of fibre

Foods high in fibre are ideal for weight control because they fill you up without adding too many kilojoules. Fruits, vegetables, legumes and wholegrain based foods are also a good source of slow release energy, reducing your body's need to store excess kilojoules. What's more, high-fibre foods offer a wide range of additional health benefits, such as reduced blood pressure and cholesterol levels and improved bowel function.

Day 33

Motivational quote of the day

'Know the true value of time; snatch, seize, and enjoy every moment of it. No idleness, no delay, no procrastination; never put off till tomorrow what you can do today.' – Earl of Chesterfield

	Planned activity	Activity journal
Beginner	Walk at level 3 (somewhat easy) for 20 minutes	
Walk Off Weight	Walk at level 4 (moderate) for 35 minutes	
Advanced	Interval training Level 7 (very hard) walk/run for 40 to 60 seconds x 15 Level 4 (moderate) walk for 60 to 80 seconds x 15	

	Menu planner	Food diary
Breakfast		
Lunch		
Dinner		
Snacks		
Glasses of water		☐☐☐☐☐☐☐☐

Trainer's notes – Practise visualisation

If your mind begins to wander during your walks, why not try some visualisation. By creating a visual image of something you want, or what you want to achieve, you will be better prepared to achieve it. By imagining yourself exercising every day, or saying no to that second glass of wine, you are helping to convince yourself that you can actually do it. Why not use your walking time more effectively by further developing your self-belief.

Day 34

Motivational quote of the day

'The most important thing to do is set goals. Training is a waste of time if you don't have goals.' – Samantha Riley

	Planned activity	Activity journal
Beginner	Walk at level 2 (very easy) for 30 minutes	
Walk Off Weight	Walk at level 5 (somewhat hard) for 25 minutes Walk at level 3 (somewhat easy) for 20 minutes	
Advanced	Strength training for 30 minutes Walk at level 6 (hard) for 20 minutes	

	Menu planner	Food diary
Breakfast		
Lunch		
Dinner		
Snacks		
Glasses of water		☐☐☐☐☐☐☐☐

Trainer's notes – Why perfectionism isn't so perfect

While I fully encourage you to strive to be your best, I recommend that you don't expect perfection, for example, setting a goal to exercise every day, and then feeling guilty when you have a day off. The pursuit of perfection is fraught with danger and motivational ups and downs. The reality is that you've exercised for 6 out of 7 days – a good achievement in anyone's books. Don't get too down about mistakes or inactive days, as they give you a great opportunity to learn.

Day 35

Motivational quote of the day

'I do not believe in a fate that falls on men however they act, but I do believe in a fate that falls on men unless they act.' – G.K. *Chesterton*

	Planned activity	Activity journal
Beginner	Walk at level 3 (somewhat easy) for 20 minutes	
Walk Off Weight	Walk at level 3 (somewhat easy) for 50 minutes	
Advanced	Rest day Level 3 (somewhat easy) walk for 30 to 60 minutes, or do a session of stretching	

	Menu planner	Food diary
Breakfast		
Lunch		
Dinner		
Snacks		
Glasses of water		☐☐☐☐☐☐☐☐

Trainer's notes – Week 5 is complete, and it's all about momentum

Now you have finished Week five, you should be developing some momentum. Momentum means that while it may have taken a tremendous amount of effort to get going initially, it then takes far less energy to keep going. The changes you make build on themselves, and the more changes you consistently make, the faster you move towards success.

Day 36

Motivational quote of the day

'Consult not your fears, but your hopes and your dreams. Think not about your frustrations, but about your unfulfilled potential. Concern yourself not with what you tried and failed in, but with what it is still possible for you to do.' – Pope John XXIII

	Planned activity	Activity journal
Beginner	Walk at level 2 (very easy) for 35 minutes	
Walk Off Weight	Walk at level 4 (moderate) for 40 minutes	
Advanced	Walk at level 6 (hard) for 40 minutes	

	Menu planner	Food diary
Breakfast		
Lunch		
Dinner		
Snacks		
Glasses of water		☐☐☐☐☐☐☐☐

Trainer's notes – Walk twice a day

Some people believe that you need to exercise twice a day to really boost your metabolism and burn fat. Obviously, walking twice a day won't hurt, but you don't need to over-complicate things. If you prefer to do 30 minutes in the morning and 30 minutes at night instead of 60 minutes in one go, it won't make much difference. The most important thing is that you do it.

Day 37

Motivational quote of the day

'I used to say, "I sure hope things will change." Then I learned that the only way things are going to change for me is when I change.'

— Jim Rohn

	Planned activity	Activity journal
Beginner	Walk at level 3 (somewhat easy) for 25 minutes	
Walk Off Weight	Walk at level 4 (moderate) for 40 minutes	
Advanced	Strength training for 30 minutes Walk at level 6 (hard) for 20 minutes	

	Menu planner	Food diary
Breakfast		
Lunch		
Dinner		
Snacks		
Glasses of water		☐☐☐☐☐☐☐☐

Trainer's notes – Don't give up when you fall down

There will always be days when you overeat, drink too much or miss the chance to walk. It happens. But it's how you respond to these days that can make all the difference. Don't use it as an excuse to quit because you had a bad day. Just try to think of a way you could prevent it, or reduce the impact next time similar circumstances arise. Then put it all behind you and go back to your program the very next day, or sooner.

Day 38

Motivational quote of the day

'Success is a journey, not only a destination. The doing is often more important than the outcome.' – Arthur Ashe

	Planned activity	Activity journal
Beginner	Walk at level 2 (very easy) for 35 minutes	
Walk Off Weight	Walk at level 5 (somewhat hard) for 25 minutes	
Advanced	Walk at level 6 (hard) for 45 to 60 minutes	

	Menu planner	Food diary
Breakfast		
Lunch		
Dinner		
Snacks		
Glasses of water		☐☐☐☐☐☐☐☐

Trainer's notes – Be wary of supermarket traps

Supermarkets and food manufacturers employ a wide range of strategies and marketing techniques to get you to buy foods you never intended to buy. Foods on special, foods kept at eye level and foods at point of sale are all designed to tempt you into parting with your hard earned dollars. Try to take a list next time you go grocery shopping, and stick to it.

Day 39

Motivational quote of the day

'There are no secrets to success. It is the result of preparation, hard work and learning from failure.' – Colin Powell

	Planned activity	Activity journal
Beginner	Walk at level 3 (somewhat easy) for 25 minutes	
Walk Off Weight	Walk at level 4 (moderate) for 40 minutes	
Advanced	Cross training (cycling, paddling, sports, running) for 40 to 60 minutes	

	Menu planner	Food diary
Breakfast		
Lunch		
Dinner		
Snacks		
Glasses of water		☐☐☐☐☐☐☐☐

Trainer's notes – Your fat cells don't care about the weather

Whether it's hot, cold, windy or there's beautiful sunshine outside – your fat cells don't really care. They will only shrink if you consistently tap into their fuel reserves. Try to have some alternative activities in mind for the days when you really don't feel like walking. If it's hot, try the local pool or air-conditioned gym, while that old exercise video could be ideal for a wet, windy or winter's day.

Day 40

Motivational quote of the day

'No matter how dark things seem to be or actually are, raise your sights and see the possibilities – always see them, for they're always there.' – Norman Vincent Peale

	Planned activity	Activity journal
Beginner	Walk at level 2 (very easy) for 35 minutes	
Walk Off Weight	Walk at level 4 (moderate) for 40 minutes	
Advanced	Interval training Find as many hills as you can during your walk, and walk as fast as you can up each one twice during a 40 minute walk	

	Menu planner	Food diary
Breakfast		
Lunch		
Dinner		
Snacks		
Glasses of water		☐☐☐☐☐☐☐☐

Trainer's notes – Don't skip meals

Skipping meals to lose weight actually makes things worse, and increases your chances of gaining weight. When you limit your kilojoule intake too drastically, the body alters its metabolism, slowing down the amount of kilojoules you burn and saves fat for essential functions. Be especially careful not to skip breakfast, which boosts your metabolism and encourages your body to burn fat.

Day 41

Motivational quote of the day

'Do not wait; the time will never be just right.' – Napoleon Hill

	Planned activity	Activity journal
Beginner	Walk at level 4 (moderate) for 15 minutes	
Walk Off Weight	Walk at level 5 (somewhat hard) for 25 minutes Walk at level 3 (somewhat easy) for 25 minutes	
Advanced	Strength training for 30 minutes Walk at level 6 (hard) for 20 minutes	

	Menu planner	Food diary
Breakfast		
Lunch		
Dinner		
Snacks		
Glasses of water		☐☐☐☐☐☐☐☐

Trainer's notes – Eat enough protein

Make sure you include plenty of protein-rich foods in your diet to help maintain your muscle mass and keep your metabolism firing. Choose your protein-rich foods wisely, as they are often accompanied by fat. Look for lean meats, low-fat dairy products, eggs (go easy on the yolks), pulses and nuts.

Day 42

Motivational quote of the day

'The ultimate measure of a man is not where he stands in moments of comfort and convenience, but where he stands at times of challenge and controversy.' – Martin Luther King Jr

	Planned activity	Activity journal
Beginner	Walk at level 2 (very easy) for 40 minutes	
Walk Off Weight	Walk at level 3 (somewhat easy) for 55 minutes	
Advanced	Rest day Level 3 (somewhat easy) walk for 30 to 60 minutes, or do a yoga class/video	

	Menu planner	Food diary
Breakfast		
Lunch		
Dinner		
Snacks		
Glasses of water		☐☐☐☐☐☐☐☐

Trainer's notes – The end of Week 6 – well done

I trust you are finding now that healthy food can still taste great. By training your taste buds, eating well can gradually transform from something you try into a new passion. Be enthusiastic about finding new recipes and learning more about the foods you put into your body. It's a worthwhile investment, and your body will thank you for it.

Day 43

Motivational quote of the day

'Everybody thinks of changing humanity, but nobody thinks of changing himself.' – Leo Tolstoy

	Planned activity	Activity journal
Beginner	Walk at level 3 (somewhat easy) for 25 minutes	
Walk Off Weight	Walk at level 4 (moderate) for 40 minutes	
Advanced	Walk at level 6 (hard) for 45 minutes	

	Menu planner	Food diary
Breakfast		
Lunch		
Dinner		
Snacks		
Glasses of water		☐☐☐☐☐☐☐☐

Trainer's notes – Dump, don't dunk your biscuits

Biscuits might seem like an easy snack, or a convenient addition to your cup of tea or coffee, but they are junk food, plain and simple. They are full of fat, sugar, salt and kilojoules, and are low in anything resembling nature or good nutrition. They can be high in trans fats, the worst kind of fat for your heart, while some popular biscuits contain more sugar than flour. Even the reduced-fat varieties are usually still high in fat and kilojoules. Fruit is a far more nutritious snack, and just as convenient. Have your cup of tea or coffee without the junk food.

Day 44

Motivational quote of the day

'He who is good at excuses is generally good for nothing else.'
— Samuel Foote

	Planned activity	Activity journal
Beginner	Walk at level 4 (moderate) for 15 minutes	
Walk Off Weight	Walk at level 4 (moderate) for 40 minutes	
Advanced	Strength training for 30 minutes Walk at level 6 (hard) for 25 minutes	

	Menu planner	Food diary
Breakfast		
Lunch		
Dinner		
Snacks		
Glasses of water		☐☐☐☐☐☐☐☐

Trainer's notes – Exercise equipment

If you are looking for some variety, or a good option for those cold, wet or miserable days, then exercise equipment can be beneficial. In addition to treadmills, other machines such as steppers and elliptical trainers can also help you burn off extra kilojoules and break up your walking routine. Exercise bikes and rowers are also beneficial, but use fewer kilojoules because the seat supports your weight.

Day 45

Motivational quote of the day

'Some people can't see the solution. Others can't see the problem.'
— G.K. Chesterton

	Planned activity	Activity journal
Beginner	Walk at level 2 (very easy) for 40 minutes	
Walk Off Weight	Walk at level 5 (somewhat hard) for 30 minutes	
Advanced	Walk at level 5 (somewhat hard) for 45 to 60 minutes	

	Menu planner	Food diary
Breakfast		
Lunch		
Dinner		
Snacks		
Glasses of water		☐☐☐☐☐☐☐☐

Trainer's notes – The low down on low GI

Eating foods with a low glycaemic index (GI) is another way to help with weight control. The GI ranks foods based on how quickly they raise blood glucose levels. Low GI foods such as legumes, skim milk, porridge and tomatoes raise blood glucose levels slowly, making them an ideal source of energy to fuel your walks.

Day 46

Motivational quote of the day

'The successful person makes a habit of doing what the failing person doesn't like to do.' – Thomas Edison

	Planned activity	Activity journal
Beginner	Walk at level 3 (somewhat easy) for 30 minutes	
Walk Off Weight	Walk at level 4 (moderate) for 40 minutes	
Advanced	Cross training (cycling, paddling, sports, running) for 40 to 60 minutes	

	Menu planner	Food diary
Breakfast		
Lunch		
Dinner		
Snacks		
Glasses of water		□ □ □ □ □ □ □ □

Trainer's notes – When to use the heart tick

Selecting foods with the National Heart Foundation's 'tick' is an easy way to make healthy food choices. Approved foods are generally lower in saturated fat, salt, sugar, and in some cases, kilojoules. However, it still pays to read the labels. Food manufacturers pay for the tick, so a competitor's product without the tick could still be a better choice.

Day 47

Motivational quote of the day

'The majority of people meet with failure because they lack the persistence to create new plans to take the place of failed plans.'
— Mark Victor Hansen

	Planned activity	Activity journal
Beginner	Walk at level 4 (moderate) for 15 minutes	
Walk Off Weight	Walk at level 4 (moderate) for 40 minutes	
Advanced	Walk at level 7 (very hard) for the distance between 3 telegraph poles, and level 4 (moderate) for the next 2 poles. Try to do 20 intervals, and finish with level 5 (somewhat hard) for 20 minutes	

	Menu planner	Food diary
Breakfast		
Lunch		
Dinner		
Snacks		
Glasses of water		☐☐☐☐☐☐☐☐

Trainer's notes – Coffee can speed up weight loss

Caffeine has been shown to stimulate the hormones involved in removing fat from the fat cells during exercise. One or two cups of black coffee before exercise will increase fat burning by delaying the use of sugar as fuel. Caffeine also increases the body's metabolic rate. Just be wary of the company that coffee keeps, such as full cream milk, cream, sugar, cakes and biscuits.

Day 48

Motivational quote of the day

'Success isn't something you chase. It is something you have to put forth the effort for constantly; then maybe it'll come when you least expect it.' – Michael Jordan

	Planned activity	Activity journal
Beginner	Walk at level 2 (very easy) for 40 minutes	
Walk Off Weight	Walk at level 5 (somewhat hard) for 30 minutes Walk at level 4 (moderate) for 20 minutes	
Advanced	Strength training for 30 minutes Walk at level 6 (hard) for 25 minutes	

	Menu planner	Food diary
Breakfast		
Lunch		
Dinner		
Snacks		
Glasses of water		☐☐☐☐☐☐☐☐

Trainer's notes – Sports drinks only useful after 90 minutes

If your goal is weight control, sports drinks are only useful if you have exercised for more than 90 minutes (60 minutes at a high intensity). Otherwise, you need the extra kilojoules like a hole in the head. Approximately 99 per cent of sweat is water, and the typical non-athlete only needs to replace the water.

Day 49

Motivational quote of the day

'In the middle of difficulty lies opportunity.' – Albert Einstein

	Planned activity	Activity journal
Beginner	Walk at level 3 (somewhat easy) for 30 minutes	
Walk Off Weight	Walk at level 3 (somewhat easy) for 60 minutes	
Advanced	Rest day Level 3 (somewhat easy) walk for 30 to 60 minutes, or do a Tai Chi class/video	

	Menu planner	Food diary
Breakfast		
Lunch		
Dinner		
Snacks		
Glasses of water		☐☐☐☐☐☐☐☐

Trainer's notes – Week 7 – you have come so far

With the finish line in sight, it's important to consider how you think about your weight and fitness. Try to look upon your health as a journey, not a destination. The changes you make to lose weight must be maintained if you want to keep the weight off. Try to focus on the process, and not the results. You can't control your results, but you can control what you do to get results. If you follow the process of healthy eating and regular activity, the results will come.

Day 50

Motivational quote of the day

'There are powers inside of you, which, if you could discover and use, would make of you everything you ever dreamed or imagined you could become.' – Orison Swett Marden

	Planned activity	Activity journal
Beginner	Walk at level 4 (moderate) for 20 minutes	
Walk Off Weight	Walk at level 4 (moderate) for 45 minutes	
Advanced	Walk at level 6 (hard) for 50 minutes	

	Menu planner	Food diary
Breakfast		
Lunch		
Dinner		
Snacks		
Glasses of water		☐☐☐☐☐☐☐☐

Trainer's notes – Juice bar warning

The liquid kilojoule bombs that juice bars disguise as health drinks can really make it hard for you to get results. People who do a big workout then guzzle down a massive glass of juice are undoing much of their good work. Your body will get little hunger satisfaction and lots of added fuel that will still have to be used up before you can burn off stored body fat. In terms of fat loss, juice bar drinks are no different to having a soft drink. Drink water, and eat fruits and vegetables instead.

Day 51

Motivational quote of the day

'Goals are new, forward-moving objectives. They magnetise you towards them.' – Mark Victor Hansen

	Planned activity	Activity journal
Beginner	Walk at level 2 (very easy) for 45 minutes	
Walk Off Weight	Walk at level 4 (moderate) for 45 minutes	
Advanced	Strength training for 30 minutes Walk at level 6 (hard) for 25 minutes	

	Menu planner	Food diary
Breakfast		
Lunch		
Dinner		
Snacks		
Glasses of water		☐ ☐ ☐ ☐ ☐ ☐ ☐ ☐

Trainer's notes – Avoid the de-motivators

In Chapter 10, I encourage you to seek out strategies that drive and motivate you towards getting results. But it's also important to avoid the things that de-motivate you. Avoid comparing your rate of loss or change to others, or spending time with toxic friends or family who are a negative influence on your results.

Day 52

Motivational quote of the day

'There is no such thing as a good excuse.' – *Dero Ames Saunders*

	Planned activity	Activity journal
Beginner	Walk at level 3 (somewhat easy) for 30 minutes	
Walk Off Weight	Walk at level 5 (somewhat hard) for 30 minutes	
Advanced	Walk at level 5 (somewhat hard) for 45 to 60 minutes	

	Menu planner	Food diary
Breakfast		
Lunch		
Dinner		
Snacks		
Glasses of water		☐☐☐☐☐☐☐☐

Trainer's notes – Eat slower to be slimmer

It's estimated to take around 20 minutes for your brain to register that your stomach is full. So by eating slower, you'll need less food (and kilojoules) to feel satisfied. Chew each mouthful thoroughly, and really savour your food. Slow eating can also help to prevent abdominal bloating.

Day 53

Motivational quote of the day

'Some men have thousands of reasons why they cannot do what they want to, when all they need is one reason why they can.'

— Mary Frances Berry

	Planned activity	Activity journal
Beginner	Walk at level 4 (moderate) for 20 minutes	
Walk Off Weight	Walk at level 4 (moderate) for 45 minutes	
Advanced	Cross training (cycling, paddling, sports, running) for 40 to 60 minutes	

	Menu planner	Food diary
Breakfast		
Lunch		
Dinner		
Snacks		
Glasses of water		☐☐☐☐☐☐☐☐

Trainer's notes – Make your home a health farm

Make sure your fridge, kitchen and food pantry all support your new, healthier lifestyle. If you don't have junk foods in your home, you are much less likely to eat them. Have tasty, healthy foods available quickly and easily, and a good supply of herbs and spices to add flavour without fat. Make sure your kitchen is well equipped with non-stick cooking pans, a microwave and a grill so you can cook up healthy and tasty meals.

Day 54

Motivational quote of the day

'Our attitudes control our lives. Attitudes are a secret power working 24 hours a day, for good or bad. It is of paramount importance that we know how to harness and control this great force.' – Tom Blandi

	Planned activity	Activity journal
Beginner	Walk at level 2 (very easy) for 45 minutes	
Walk Off Weight	Walk at level 5 (somewhat hard) for 35 minutes	
Advanced	Find the biggest flight of stairs near you, and walk as fast as you can 2 steps at a time. Repeat for 20 minutes, then finish with level 4 (moderate) for 20 minutes	

	Menu planner	Food diary
Breakfast		
Lunch		
Dinner		
Snacks		
Glasses of water		☐☐☐☐☐☐☐☐

Trainer's notes – Reward yourself

When you've reached a goal, small or large, you deserve a treat. Knowing there is a reward to be gained reinforces your new behaviour, and helps to drive you towards taking action. Aim for fortnightly or monthly rewards that keep you focused, such as walking six days a week for four weeks. Choose non-food related rewards that won't blow all your good work, such as having a massage, or buying a new book or CD.

Day 55

Motivational quote of the day

'We must either find a way or make one.' – Hannibal

	Planned activity	Activity journal
Beginner	Walk at level 3 (somewhat easy) for 30 minutes	
Walk Off Weight	Walk at level 6 (hard) for 20 minutes Walk at level 4 (moderate) for 30 minutes	
Advanced	Strength training for 30 minutes Walk at level 6 (hard) for 25 minutes	

	Menu planner	Food diary
Breakfast		
Lunch		
Dinner		
Snacks		
Glasses of water		☐☐☐☐☐☐☐☐

Trainer's notes – Stay well informed

It really helps to stay up-to-date with any new information and research on health, fitness and weight control. New studies are released almost daily that recommend new strategies, confirm old ones, and dispel myths and misunderstandings. One way you can do this is to subscribe to my free weekly email tip: The Better Body Update.

Just go to my website at www.andrewcate.com

Day 56

Motivational quote of the day

'There's only one way to succeed in anything, and that is to give everything.' – *Vince Lombardi*

	Planned activity	Activity journal
Beginner	Walk at level 4 (moderate) for 20 minutes	
Walk Off Weight	Walk at level 3 (somewhat easy) for 60 minutes	
Advanced	Rest day Level 3 (somewhat easy) walk for 30 to 60 minutes, or do a Pilates class/video	

	Menu planner	Food diary
Breakfast		
Lunch		
Dinner		
Snacks		
Glasses of water		☐ ☐ ☐ ☐ ☐ ☐ ☐ ☐

Trainer's notes – Congratulations – you have finished the 8-week challenge

What a great achievement. I knew you could do it! Hopefully, you have lost weight, feel fitter, and have started to make walking a habit. So where to now? If you were a beginner, move on to the Walk Off Weight program. If you have completed the Walk Off Weight program, and want to ramp things up, it's time to try the advanced program. Just read Chapter 9 first. If you have just completed the advanced program, you now have a good record of your last 8 weeks' activity. This can serve as a great benchmark for your next 8 weeks' activity, as you have times, distances and intensities to improve upon.

8

The Walk Off Weight recipes

So what can I eat?

Food is a very personal thing, and I don't believe there is a perfect, single diet out there for everyone. People have different tastes and reasons for eating, and there needs to be flexibility if people are going to stick with a healthy-eating plan. It should take time to modify or change the way you eat, otherwise, you will just want to go back to the way you ate before. But I will say that if you want to lose weight and body fat, there are some foods you should eat more of, and some you should eat less of. You saw in Chapter 6 my list of 10 fat-storing foods to cut back on. Now it's time to look at some specific foods to eat more of. My 10 fat-burning power foods should be the foundation of your diet. They really help to accelerate fat loss, and are the basis of many of the recipes and fast feast ideas that follow.

 ### The 10 fat-burning power foods

1 Beans, peas and lentils (legumes)
2 Wholegrains
3 Water-rich vegetables
4 Berries
5 Fish and seafood
6 Lean meats
7 Nuts and seeds
8 Skim milk smoothies
9 Eggs
10 Soy products

Recipes to change your diet, and your weight

I find the most practical way to help people modify the way they eat is to work on individual meals. Nearly all of us have breakfast, lunch, dinner and snacks in some form or another. I have broken the recipes up into those 4 categories to keep things simple. Just like your walking, take one step at a time, and gradually build up your repertoire of healthy meals and snacks.

Incorporate some of these recipes and fast feast ideas into your meals over the course of your 8-week challenge. My hope is that some of these recipes and fast feast ideas will become part of your new foundation for lifelong healthy eating. These recipes can help you stick to the healthy-eating strategies I have outlined in Chapter 6. If you can be patient and positive while eating fewer kilojoules and eating more healthily, you can lose weight, and still enjoy your food.

Breakfast

A good breakfast has long been recommended for weight loss and good health, yet it is the meal most likely to be missed. It doesn't make sense to avoid food when you have just gone 8 to 10 hours without eating or drinking. A healthy breakfast will give you energy and re-hydrate your body. If you're short on time in the mornings, there is a wide range of easy to eat foods you can choose from. Take a closer look at the fast feast ideas on page 118. Many of the following breakfast recipes that follow don't take long to prepare.

Breakfast cereals

While breakfast cereals can be a tasty, healthy and easy start to the day, there is a wide gap between types when it comes to nutritional quality. Choose a cereal that is low in fat, salt and sugar, and high in complex carbohydrate and dietary fibre. Avoid full cream milk on your cereal, as this can give you over 10 grams of unhealthy saturated fat to start the day. If you enjoy sugary cereals, mix them with a high-fibre cereal. When considering commercial breakfast cereals, check the nutritional information table to see if they meet the following criteria:

Per 100g serving	
Fat	5 grams or less
Sugar	10 grams or less
Fibre	4 grams or more
Sodium	250mg or less

Cereals that normally meet these criteria include wheat biscuits, natural muesli, oat or wheat bran, shredded wheat and bran flakes.

RECIPE

Easy breakfast mix (serves 5 to 7)

3 wheat biscuits, crushed
1 cup sweet cereal (honey wheat puffs, crunchy nut cornflakes)
1 cup low-fibre cereal (rice bubbles, corn flakes)
½ cup rolled oats
½ cup breakfast sprinkle (nut, seed and dried fruit mix)
¼ cup bran (rice, oat, psyllium, wheat bran or wheatgerm)

Mix all the ingredients together in an airtight container.

Variation – *You can substitute or add lots of other cereals in the recipe, such as bran flakes, Sultana Bran or shredded wheat. Add skim milk, fresh fruit and low-fat yoghurt.*

 Fat-burning power food – Wholegrains

Many white or processed carbohydrate foods use only the kilojoule-containing component of the grain (the endosperm), removing the outer bran layer and the germ. The manufacturer takes out the fibre, healthy fats, antioxidants, vitamins and goodness, and you get the kilojoules. Wholegrains contain all the original parts of the grain seed, just as nature intended. They fill you up more, are a better source of energy, and help prevent disease and illness. So look for wholemeal pasta, brown rice and multigrain bread. Other choices include barley, buckwheat, bulgur, corn, oats, rye, quinoa, sorghum, spelt and wild rice. Just don't go overboard with your portions of these foods, as they are kilojoule dense. Aim for 2 to 4 servings a day.

Toast

Toast is probably the easiest breakfast food you can make, but your selection of bread, the spread and topping you use can vary the health benefits of toast dramatically.

- **Bread** – Bread is a high-kilojoule food, yet it can provide fullness and nutrition, or fat-storing excess depending on the choices you make. Wholegrain varieties of bread are by far and away the best choice, because they are much higher in fibre. It's more filling, so you need fewer kilojoules to feel satisfied. The fibre also slows down its absorption, so it's a better source of long-term energy, and it reduces the need for insulin, which in turn prevents fat storage. Wholemeal is the next best choice, because it has wholegrains, even if they have been ground up. This would speed up the rate of absorption compared to wholegrains left as nature intended. Next on the list is high-fibre white bread, which is a good choice for kids who won't eat multigrain or wholemeal. Finally, and way down the list, is white bread. It has less than half the fibre content of multigrain bread, and is also lower in vitamins and minerals. It is a fat-storing food, so avoid it like the plague.

- **Spreads** – Butter and margarine are fat-storing foods. Eliminate them, or minimise their use.

- **Toppings** – Common spreads like jam, marmalade and honey are very high in easily digestible sugars, so don't spread them too thickly. Vegemite is high in some vitamins, but most people would not enjoy it without butter. Try using cottage cheese instead. Peanut butter is high in fat, but the fats are mostly healthy, so enjoy in moderation. Finally, chocolate spreads are high in fat and sugar, so keep them to a minimum.

-- (**RECIPE**)

French toast (serves 1)

1 egg white
1 tablespoon skim milk
¼ teaspoon nutmeg
1 slice multigrain bread
½ a small banana
1 teaspoon honey

1. *Whisk the egg white, milk and nutmeg in a small bowl.*

2. *Soak the bread in the egg mixture.*

3. *Heat a non-stick cooking pan on a medium to high heat, and cover lightly with cooking spray. Brown the bread on both sides for about 2 to 3 minutes per side until golden.*

4. *Top with sliced banana and a drizzle of honey.*

Variation – You can also top the French toast with chopped strawberries and a little maple syrup.

Fat-burning power food – Skim milk smoothies

I just love smoothies. They are a wonderful, tasty and healthy way to start the day. You can have them for breakfast, or as a healthy snack. This banana berry recipe is one of my favourites, and contains three fat-burning power foods. The milk gives you protein, the fruit gives you sweetness and the psyllium husks give you fullness. Smoothies certainly taste better than a protein bar, and match up nutritionally with most powdered protein supplements. What's more, they are significantly cheaper. Using low-fat dairy products, such as skim milk, is essential as it significantly reduces the kilojoule content. Full-fat milk, yoghurt or ice cream would cancel out any benefit. With all the extra ingredients, smoothies still taste great with skim milk. Just make sure you keep your portions under control.

(**RECIPE**)

Banana berry smoothie (serves 1 to 2)

250 ml skim milk
2 tablespoons low-fat yoghurt
1 small banana
⅓ cup frozen berries
1 teaspoon honey
2 ice cubes
1 tablespoon psyllium husks (optional)

1. *Combine all the ingredients in a blender and process until smooth and frothy.*
2. *Serve in a chilled milkshake glass.*

Hint – *If you semi-freeze your banana for about an hour, your smoothie will be even creamier. Just make sure to peel the skin off first, and break the banana into a few pieces before placing it in a plastic bag or small container. Let the psyllium husks soak in the milk for a few minutes so they soften.*

Variation – *Combine your favourite ingredients using the list of creative additions on the following page to make your own favourite smoothie.*

Fruits	Dairy and alternatives	Extras
Berries, banana, strawberries, mango, passion fruit, peach, apricot, pear, pineapple. Fresh, frozen, or canned fruits can all be used.	Skim milk, low-fat soy milk, rice milk, low-fat yoghurt, frozen low-fat yoghurt, light custard, skim milk powder, low-fat ice cream, light evaporated milk, soy powder, whey powder.	Ice cubes, oats, oatmeal, wheatgerm, honey, malt powder, Ovaltine, diet caramel topping, vanilla essence, raw egg whites, nutmeg, all spice, cinnamon.

 Fat-burning power food – Ultimate oats

One of the easiest, cheapest and healthiest ways to eat more wholegrains is to have oats. Being a wholegrain, they are fat-burning power food. They are a good source of fibre, protein, vitamins, minerals and healthy fats. Just avoid the commercial toasted mueslis, which are baked in fat. Eaten as muesli in summer, porridge in winter, or even added to soups and smoothies, they are versatile and delicious. Why not try these muesli recipes and see for yourself?

RECIPE

Soft Swiss muesli (serves 2–4)

½ cup rolled oats
½ cup skim milk
200 ml low-fat yoghurt
½ green apple, cored and grated (skin on)
2 tablespoons sultanas
½ teaspoon ground cinnamon
2 tablespoons slivered almonds
1 tablespoon sunflower kernels

1. *Combine the oats, milk, yoghurt, apple, sultanas, and cinnamon in a large bowl. Cover and refrigerate overnight. The next morning, sprinkle the almonds and seeds over the oats mixture just prior to eating.*

Hint – *If you like your muesli thick, use a little less milk. If you like it thinner, add some extra skim milk or low-fat soy milk at Step 1. You can also add a little honey if you like a little more sweetness.*

Variation – *This recipe is only limited by your imagination. You can add different types of nuts and seeds. You can also substitute or add virtually any fruit you like instead of the apple.*

Natural muesli (serves 4 to 6)

1 cup rolled oats
¼ cup unprocessed bran
¼ cup sultanas
¼ cup chopped, dried apricots
¼ cup chopped almonds
2 tablespoons sunflower kernels
1 tablespoon sesame seeds
1 teaspoon ground cinnamon

Mix all the ingredients together and store in an airtight container. There is enough to last 1 person for 1 week.

Hint – *If you are in a rush, you can have this with yoghurt instead of skim milk, and eat it on the run.*

Variation – *You can use different or additional grains, such as rolled barley, quinoa, rolled rye or wheatgerm. You can also try different nuts and seeds, such as walnuts, pecans, macadamias, pistachios, pumpkin seeds or sesame seeds, and a small amount of shredded coconut or dried fruits.*

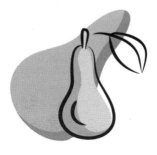

The weekend breakfast

I like to vary my breakfast on the weekend, when I have a little more time for preparation. I encourage you to avoid the typical high-fat breakfast foods such as bacon, fried eggs, hash browns and sausages. These are not only loaded with kilojoules, they also make you more likely to reach for a mid-morning snack. You can still enjoy a hearty, hot breakfast without all the fat, as you will see with the following two easy recipes.

RECIPE

Cooked breakfast

1 boiled egg
⅓ cup baked beans
½ tomato, dry-fried
2 slices lean ham
1 slice multigrain toast (no butter)
pepper to taste

1. *Boil a saucepan of water, and cook your egg to the desired level of hardness. (See hint below.)*

2. *In a non-stick pan, heat the ham, tomato and baked beans.*

3. *Serve over multigrain toast, and top with cracked pepper if desired.*

Hint – *Bring eggs to room temperature before using. When the water is boiling gently, carefully lower the egg into the water, and start timing from when the water re-boils. Timing depends on the size and degree of hardness desired. Generally it's 3 to 4 and a half minutes for soft-boiled, 4 and a half to 6 minutes for medium-boiled and 6 to 7 minutes for hard-boiled.*

Variation – *Other tasty additions and substitutions for a healthy, hot breakfast include poached eggs, scrambled eggs using two egg whites, one yolk and skim milk, grilled mushrooms, steamed spinach, asparagus and smoked salmon.*

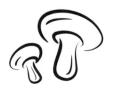

Ham and tomato omelette (serves 1)

1 whole egg
1 egg white
1 tablespoon skim milk
½ teaspoon paprika
¼ cup chopped tomatoes
¼ cup lean ham, sliced
1 teaspoon chopped fresh parsley
pepper to taste

1. *Combine the egg, egg white, skim milk and paprika together in bowl until the yolk is mixed in well.*
2. *Add the tomatoes, ham and parsley to the egg mixture.*
3. *Lightly spray a non-stick fry pan with cooking oil, and pre-warm it to a medium heat.*
4. *Pour the mixture into pan, and cook until the mixture sets.*
5. *Serve over one slice of multigrain toast, and season with pepper to taste.*

Hint – *Put a saucepan lid over the pan to speed up the cooking process and prevent the bottom from burning.*

Variation – *There are many things you can add to an omelette, such as extra herbs (basil, oregano, thyme), water-rich vegetables (chopped capsicum, asparagus, shallots, grated zucchini), and different meats, such as smoked salmon, canned tuna or shredded chicken.*

 Fat-burning power food – Eggs

Breakfast is a great time to enjoy eggs, which are highly nutritious and filling, and contain more protein per gram than any other food. They are high in cholesterol, but this is only a problem if you have existing high blood cholesterol levels. If your blood cholesterol levels are within the healthy range, and you limit other saturated fats in the diet, then 5 to 7 eggs a week should be fine. Another concern is the company eggs keep, such as oil, butter, salt, sausages, bacon, hollandaise sauce and hash browns. Go easy on the extras. Of course, you can eat as many egg whites as you like. It's only the yolk that has fat or cholesterol.

Fast feast breakfast ideas

- Fruit such as apples, bananas, strawberries, pears and mandarins are not messy, and can be virtually eaten on the run.
- A fruit salad can make a tasty, easy breakfast.
- Grab a drinking yoghurt and a low-fat muesli bar on the way out the door.
- Commercial breakfast drinks and smoothies are a quick and easy option (if you don't have time to make your own).
- Toast a wholegrain English muffin and top with peanut butter and honey.
- If you don't like traditional breakfast foods such as cereal or toast, eat something else that you enjoy. Try sandwiches, creamed rice, pasta or casserole if it means you will eat something, and take advantage of all the benefits associated with eating a healthy breakfast.
- Top some pancakes (made with wholemeal flour, egg whites and skim milk) with strawberries and low-fat yoghurt.
- Bake some low-fat muffins with bran (or wholemeal flour), fruit and low-fat yoghurt, and freeze them. You can then defrost them each morning in the microwave one by one over the next week or two.
- The recipes for snacks listed later in this chapter could also make a good breakfast.

Lunch

After you have used up all of the fuel from your morning meal, it's important to eat something healthy. The longer you wait, the more likely you will be to crave junk. A healthy lunch can also give you energy, preventing you from feeling sluggish throughout the afternoon. It doesn't need to be a huge meal, otherwise you might end up feeling like a siesta. Ideally, include a quality wholegrain type food, a low-fat protein-based food, and some fibrous vegetables.

Light salads

Salads are a tasty way to include lots of vegetables, legumes and lean meats in your diet while helping to keep your kilojoule intake down. You can practically live on them in the warmer months. They are great for lunch, side dishes or a light dinner, and you can make up a large bowl to keep you going for a couple of days. Always look to add different vegetables, herbs, nuts and even fruits. Be creative. Try to stick with low-kilojoule dressings and vinaigrettes that rely on a small amount of good quality oil. Vinegars, lemon juice, lime juice, wine, tomato juice, and fruit juices are a great way to bring out the flavour of your salads. Give high-kilojoule additions the flick, like creamy dressings, mayonnaise, fatty meats, cheese and too much oil.

RECIPE

Tuna salad (serves 4)

½ small red onion, finely diced
½ cup cherry tomatoes, halved
½ cup green beans, chopped
¼ cup canned white beans (cannellini), drained
½ red (or yellow) capsicum, roughly chopped
2 tablespoons fresh parsley, chopped
400g fillet-style tuna, drained
pepper to taste

Dressing
2 teaspoons lemon juice
¼ cup low-fat natural yoghurt
1 tablespoon extra virgin olive oil
1 teaspoon sugar

1. *Combine the onion, tomatoes, green beans, white beans, capsicum and parsley in large bowl.*

2. *Gently stir through the tuna and top with cracked pepper if desired.*

3. *Add the lemon juice, yoghurt, oil and sugar to a small bowl, and mix well. Pour over the salad and serve immediately.*

Hint – *You can actually serve this as a warm salad. Microwave on high for two minutes. Drain off any liquid before adding the dressing.*

Variation – *You can have this salad on its own, or use it as a topping over brown rice, wholemeal pasta or a small baked potato. Other vegetables that you could substitute or add include cucumbers, shallots, steamed asparagus spears or steamed sweet potato.*

Chicken Caesar salad (serves 2)

2 chicken tenderloins, cut into thirds lengthways
2 slices lean ham, cut into strips
6 asparagus spears, blanched
1 cos lettuce, leaves separated
½ cup cherry tomatoes, halved
1 slice multigrain bread, crust removed, toasted then cubed
1 teaspoon grated parmesan cheese

Dressing
1 tablespoon low-fat mayonnaise
2 tablespoons low-fat natural yoghurt
1 teaspoon wholegrain mustard
salt and pepper to taste

1. *Heat a non-stick frying pan over medium heat. Spray with cooking spray, and add the chicken. Stir until cooked, then set aside.*

2. *Spray the pan again, and add the ham. Heat for 1 to 2 minutes, then set aside.*

3. *Boil, steam or microwave the asparagus until just tender. Drain and rinse under cold water.*

4. *Arrange the lettuce, asparagus, tomatoes and bread cubes in a serving bowl. Scatter with chicken and ham and top with parmesan cheese.*

5. *To make the dressing, combine the mayonnaise, yoghurt, mustard and seasoning in a small bowl. Drizzle over salad.*

Hint – *You can grill the chicken breasts and ham as an alternative to frying.*

Variation – *You can add anchovies to this recipe if you enjoy them. Chopped semi-dried tomatoes, blanched snow peas and grilled capsicum also work well.*

Sandwiches and beyond

There are significant benefits for your weight and your wallet from making a healthy sandwich for lunch. They are quick and convenient, but the challenge is to keep them tasty and interesting. If you get bored with bread or the same old meats, it might be time for a sandwich makeover. You can mix and match the sandwich ingredients from the table below for a great lunch, or try one of the tasty recipes that follow. If you don't have time to make your own, you will usually find these ingredients at most sandwich bars.

Bread	Flavourings	Protein food	Vegetables	Others
multigrain rolls	low-fat mayonnaise	tuna	lettuce	mashed banana
wholemeal sliced	herbs (fresh and dried)	salmon	sprouts	grated apple
multigrain sliced	spices	baked beans	carrot	grated pear
high-fibre white	mustard	cottage cheese	celery	sultanas
Lebanese bread	pickles and relish	ricotta cheese	tomato	dried apricots
pita bread	chutney	low-fat cheese slices	onion	dried apple
lavash (flat) bread	hummus	low-fat sliced meats	capsicum	pineapple
mountain (flat) bread	apple sauce	shredded chicken	mushroom	
cracker breads	Vegemite	hard-boiled egg	beetroot	
tortillas	baba ghanoush	peanut butter	avocado	

-- (**RECIPE**)

Chicken salad wrap (serves 1)

1 flour tortilla
⅓ cup shredded chicken breast
¼ cup tomato, diced
¼ cup carrot, grated
¼ small avocado
1 tablespoon low-fat mayonnaise
2 lettuce leaves

1. *Microwave the tortilla for 15 seconds on high.*
2. *Spread the chicken, tomato, carrot, avocado, mayonnaise and lettuce down the centre of the warm tortilla.*
3. *Fold two opposite sides toward centre, and roll up the tortilla from an open end. Cut the wrap in half, and cover each half in grease proof paper. Serve immediately or refrigerate until ready to serve.*

(RECIPE)

Warm roast beef and avocado roll (serves 1)

1 multigrain roll
2 slices of rare roast beef
2 to 4 thin slices red onion
¼ avocado
2 teaspoons fruit chutney
½ small tomato, sliced
½ teaspoon paprika

1. *Cut the roll through the centre.*

2. *Distribute the remaining ingredients evenly over the two portions of the roll.*

3. *Heat in the microwave for 20 to 30 seconds on high until the roll is warm. Serve immediately.*

Hint – *You can also grill this in the oven if you like your bread a little crusty.*

 ## *Fat-burning power food – Beans, peas and lentils (legumes)*

Legumes are high in protein and quality carbohydrates, low in fat, have no cholesterol, and are packed with fibre. Legumes are the ideal fat-burning, high-energy food, as they regulate blood sugar and insulin levels, providing maximum fullness for minimum kilojoules. They are the ultimate low-GI food, making you feel fuller for longer. Try to include beans, peas and lentils in at least 2 to 4 meals each week.

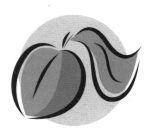

Soups

One of the best ways to lose weight is to eat lots of soup. Ideal for lunch, dinner or even as a snack, a thick, hearty soup can be very satisfying, yet very low in kilojoules. Soup is low in kilojoules because of its high water content, yet it's usually served hot, so people tend to eat it slowly and feel full afterwards. In fact, whole diet books have been devoted to soup. Load your soups up with plenty of fat-burning power foods such as vegetables, lean meats and wholegrains, and lots of flavour with herbs, spices and condiments. Avoid cream-based soups that are loaded with fat and kilojoules. Soups are also a great time saver, because you can make large batches, and reheat it quickly, or freeze the leftovers. Here are two of my favourite soup recipes.

--(*RECIPE*)

Minestrone soup (serves 4 to 6)

1 onion, chopped
2 teaspoons minced garlic
1 stick celery, chopped
½ cup green beans, chopped
2 medium carrots, chopped
3 cups water
3 beef stock cubes
1 x 410g can chopped tomatoes
1 x 410g can butter beans, drained
1 cup diced sweet potato
salt and pepper to taste

1. *In a large pot, add the onion, garlic, celery, green beans, carrots and water, and stir through the stock cubes.*

2. *Add the tomatoes, beans and sweet potato, and bring to the boil.*

3. *Simmer for 1 hour, ensuring the sweet potato is cooked through.*

Hint – *If you don't have peeled tomatoes, chopped tomatoes or even a tomato pasta sauce will work fine. You can also try commercial stock instead of water and stock cubes.*

Variation – *You can add or substitute all sorts of vegetables, legumes and grain foods in this recipe. Zucchini, spinach, squash, potato, cabbage, kidney beans, barley and cooked wholegrain pasta all work well.*

Pumpkin and sweet potato soup (serves 4 to 6)

1 onion, chopped
1 tablespoon crushed garlic
500g pumpkin, peeled and cut into large chunks
500g sweet potato, peeled and cut into large chunks
2 cups stock
3 tablespoons chopped parsley
1 cup skim milk
pepper to taste

1. *Sauté the onion and garlic with a little water in large saucepan on a medium heat until the onion is transparent.*

2. *Add the pumpkin, sweet potato and stock, and bring to the boil. Reduce heat and cover. Simmer until the pumpkin and sweet potato are tender.*

3. *Remove from the heat and add the parsley, milk and pepper, stirring through.*

4. *When the mixture cools, purée in food processor or blender. The soup is then ready to be reheated and served.*

Hint *– Serve with a crusty multigrain roll.*

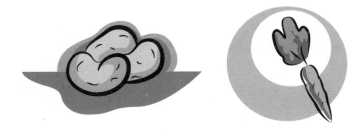

Leftovers

With time in short supply these days, it makes sense to minimise your food preparation and cooking time. By using your freezer, fast food can still be good food. Knowing you have a healthy, tasty meal available for a quick reheat at home can reduce your reliance on fast take-away junk. Foods such as lean meats, tomato-based sauces, soups and rice all freeze well. Why not spend part of your weekend making double batches of stir-fries, pastas and mixed vegetables for the week ahead. Whenever I steam some rice, I always freeze the leftovers so I can whip together this quick fried rice recipe. It doesn't take long to cook, and makes a great lunchtime meal. You can even make it for dinner, then have the leftovers for lunch the next day.

-- **RECIPE**

Fried rice (serves 4)

1 whole egg
1 egg white
1 onion, finely diced
½ cup celery, chopped
½ cup green peas (frozen)
1 red capsicum, seeded and diced
¼ cup chopped lean ham
4 shallots (spring onions), chopped
2 cups cooked brown rice
1 tablespoon soy sauce
1 tablespoon plum sauce

1. *Lightly spray a non-stick fry pan with cooking oil, and pre-warm it to a low heat.*

2. *Whisk the whole egg and egg white together, and pour mixture into pan. Cook until the mixture sets, then remove from the pan and set aside.*

3. *Add the onion, celery, peas and capsicum to the pan, and stir fry for 3 to 4 minutes.*

4. *Add the ham, shallots, rice and soy sauce and plum sauce, mixing all the ingredients together and heating through.*

5. *Gently stir through the reserved egg and serve.*

Variation – *You can add or substitute many things in your fridge or pantry in this recipe. If you have some left over meat such as chicken or pork, use it instead of the ham. If you have some corn in the pantry, that will go well, as will other vegetables such as grated carrot, chopped zucchini, or leek.*

Fast feast lunch ideas

- **Chicken salad** – Grill strips of chicken marinated in Hoisin sauce. Add to a green salad with lettuce, cherry tomatoes, sliced cucumber and cottage cheese, drizzled with balsamic vinegar.
- **Chickpea salad** – Use canned chickpeas in a green salad, dressed with a mustard, white wine and lemon juice dressing.
- **Ham and hummus wrap** – Spread hummus, sweet chilli sauce, lean ham, tomato and shredded lettuce on lavash (flat) bread, and eat rolled up.
- **Banana dog** – On a wholemeal hot dog roll, add a whole banana with cottage cheese, creamed honey and cinnamon.
- **Salmon and avocado crackers** – On a multigrain cracker bread, add smoked or canned salmon, avocado, tomato and fruit chutney.
- **Turkey and cranberry salad** – Make an easy salad using lettuce leaves, sliced turkey breast, cottage cheese, dried cranberries and snow pea sprouts.
- **Chicken and tomato salsa** – Spoon a commercial bruschetta or salsa over a grilled chicken breast, and serve with a green salad.
- **Creamy corn soup** – In a pot, add chopped ham, ½ cup water, some chopped mushroom, shallots, pepper and a small tin of creamed corn for a fast and tasty soup.

Dinner

As I mentioned in Chapter 6, it's important to minimise the portion size of your evening meal. Your activity levels and metabolic rate are winding down, so try to keep your kilojoule intake down as well. It just doesn't make sense to eat your largest meal at night. A good guide for the evening meal is to have half your plate made up of vegetables, a quarter made up from lean meat, seafood or beans, and the other quarter made up of quality carbohydrates such as brown rice, wholemeal pasta or multigrain bread. If you are sharing dinner with a partner, women need to eat a smaller portion than men. Women in general have less muscle mass, so they need fewer kilojoules to meet their daily needs.

Hot and spicy

Diets high in chilli and other spicy foods are known to bring about a slight boost in metabolic rate, helping you to burn more kilojoules. Studies have even shown that people who eat chilli regularly sleep better and rise more energetically. That can make you more likely to want to exercise. Just don't blow all those benefits by having your spicy food with a high-fat curry loaded with coconut cream. Below are two tasty, spicy recipes that won't blow your fat budget.

Chilli con carne (serves 4 to 6)

1 onion, chopped
2 teaspoons minced garlic
1 teaspoon vegetable oil
500g lean beef mince
1 x 425g can chopped tomatoes
1 x 425g can red kidney beans, drained
⅓ cup tomato paste
1 cup stock (beef, chicken or vegetable)
1 to 2 teaspoons chilli powder
½ teaspoon ground cumin
½ teaspoon paprika

1. *Add the onion and garlic to a little water in a non-stick pan on a high heat. Cook until the onion softens and the water evaporates.*

2. *Add the oil and mince meat, stirring until the meat is browned.*

3. *Add the tomatoes, beans, tomato paste, stock, chilli powder, cumin and paprika, stirring thoroughly.*

4. *Bring to the boil, then reduce heat and simmer for 5 to 10 minutes, stirring occasionally.*

Hint *– For dinner, serve with steamed vegetables and a small serving of a carbohydrate-based food, such as a baked potato, brown rice or polenta. As a lunch, serve on its own, wrapped in a tortilla, or with multigrain toast and a green salad.*

Variation *– This is chilli con carne in its most basic form, but you can add extra vegetables (corn, celery, grated carrot, capsicum, shallots) and herbs (basil, parsley, rosemary, chives). If you don't like your food too spicy, substitute the chilli powder for sweet chilli sauce, or eliminate the chilli completely. Alternatively, if you like it hot, add a little extra chilli powder, or Tabasco sauce.*

Chicken vegetable curry (serves 4 to 6)

1 onion, chopped
2 teaspoons minced garlic
500g diced chicken breast
2 tablespoons curry paste
1 carrot, diced
1 red capsicum, seeded and diced
1 cup frozen peas
1 cup diced zucchini
2 tablespoons tomato sauce
2 teaspoons fresh basil, chopped
1 x 375ml can light evaporated milk

1. *Add the onion and garlic to a little water in a non-stick pan on a high heat. Cook until the onion softens and the water evaporates.*

2. *Add the curry paste, chicken, carrot and capsicum, stirring until the meat is browned. There should be enough oil in the curry paste to prevent the chicken from sticking to the pan. Use a little water if required.*

3. *Add the peas, zucchini, tomato sauce and basil, and mix well.*

4. *Reduce the heat, and pour in the evaporated milk a little at a time, stirring constantly. Try not to let it boil intensely, as the milk can burn.*

5. *Allow to simmer gently for 10 minutes, stirring regularly.*

6. *Serve with steamed vegetables, and a small amount of brown rice.*

Hint – *If the curry is too runny, thicken it with a tablespoon of corn flour, whisking it through quickly. If you don't have curry paste, you can use curry powder with a little vegetable oil.*

Variation – *You can use different lean meats for this dish, such as beef or lamb. Other vegetables that can be used in a curry like this include cauliflower, corn and green beans. Other ways to add flavour and aroma to a curry include using additional fresh herbs such as coriander, dried spices like cumin and paprika, or other ingredients such as chopped nuts, fish sauce, lemon zest, bay leaves or kaffir lime leaves.*

Meat and vegetables

It doesn't get any better for fat and weight loss than to feast on meat and vegetables. These fat-burning power foods should make up three quarters of your evening meal. The vegetables are rich in essential nutrients such as vitamins, minerals and antioxidants, and add colour and variety to your diet. The meat gives you protein, but is also high in iron, which helps to maintain your energy levels and helps you walk with enthusiasm and vitality.

(*RECIPE*)

Garlic lamb and vegetable kebabs (makes 4 kebabs)

2 teaspoons minced garlic
2 tablespoons soy sauce
1 teaspoon oil
1 lamb backstrap, cut into cubes
1 small yellow (or red) capsicum, cut into squares
1 zucchini, cut into 1cm discs
12 cherry tomatoes
1 small red onion, cut into wedges

1. *In a small bowl, mix together the garlic, soy sauce and olive oil. Add the lamb and turn until the meat is coated in the garlic mixture. Cover and stand for 30 minutes, or refrigerate overnight. There will be more flavour if you marinate it overnight.*

2. *Thread the lamb onto the skewers, alternating with 2 vegetables at a time. Distribute the vegetables evenly over the 4 skewers.*

3. *Heat a hot plate or barbecue grill to a moderately hot temperature, and spray with cooking oil. Cook the kebabs for 5 to 8 minutes depending on how you like the lamb cooked. Turn occasionally, and serve immediately.*

Hint – *If you use wooden skewers, soak them in water for 30 minutes beforehand to prevent them from burning.*

Variation – *Other vegetables that work well with kebabs include slender eggplants, carrots and mushrooms. Other meats that would work well with this recipe include beef, veal and pork.*

Italian chicken and vegetables (serves 4)

1 onion, chopped
2 teaspoons minced garlic
1 teaspoon vegetable oil
2 chicken breasts, cubed
½ cup broccoli florets
½ cup carrot, chopped
1 red (or yellow) capsicum, roughly chopped
1 jar pasta sauce
½ cup mushrooms, chopped
2 tablespoons fresh basil, chopped
1 teaspoon paprika
pepper to taste

1. *Add the onion and garlic to a little water in a non-stick pan on a high heat. Cook until the onion softens and the water evaporates.*

2. *Add the oil, chicken breasts, broccoli, carrot and red capsicum, stirring until the meat is browned.*

3. *Add the pasta sauce, mushrooms, basil, paprika and pepper and bring to the boil, stirring thoroughly.*

4. *Reduce heat and simmer for 5 minutes, stirring occasionally.*

Variation – *You can grill the whole chicken breast, and make a sauce out of the remaining ingredients. You can then pour the sauce over the chicken breast and serve with a little brown rice. A sprinkling of cashews also works well with this dish.*

 Fat-burning power food – Lean meats

Lean meat is an ideal source of protein, which fills you up and protects your muscle tissue when you reduce your kilojoule intake. Look for lean cuts of beef, veal, kangaroo, lamb and pork. Remove the skin from chicken and turkey, and try to choose the white meat such as the breast rather than the darker meat on the thighs and legs. Trimming meats of fat and removing the skin on poultry significantly reduces their kilojoule content, and changes the food from a fat-storing food into a fat burner. Animal fats that often accompany meats are the worst type of fat for your heart, and the most likely type of fat you will store. Grill or stir fry meat with minimal oil, and use lots of herbs, spices and marinades to add flavour and taste. Tofu is a reasonable alternative if you are a vegetarian.

Stir fries

Asian stir fries are a tasty way to include lean meats and a wider variety of vegetables in your diet. A good stir fry recipe seems to bring out the best in most vegetables, and dramatically enhances their flavour. Cooking the vegetables quickly over high heat helps to keep them crisp while retaining nutrients. Boost the flavour of your stir fries with small amounts of strongly flavoured ingredients, including garlic, ginger, soy sauce, oyster sauce, fish sauce, Hoi sin sauce, plum sauce, white wine, Teriyaki marinade, honey and chilli. Try to bulk up your stir fries up with lots of water-rich vegetables, and keep your white rice intake to a minimum.

RECIPE

Sesame pork and noodle stir fry (serves 4 to 6)

250g pack of fresh rice noodles
1 onion, chopped
1 teaspoon crushed garlic
1 teaspoon sesame oil
250g lean pork, cubed
1 tablespoon light soy sauce
1 red capsicum, seeded and chopped
2 sticks celery, sliced
2 cups button mushrooms, halved
¼ cup shallots, chopped
1 tablespoon sesame seeds
2 tablespoons Hoisin sauce
1 tablespoon fish sauce

1. *Boil the noodles as directed, drain and set aside.*
2. *Add the onion and garlic to a little water in a non-stick pan on a high heat. Cook until the onion softens and the water evaporates.*
3. *Add the oil and pork and stir until the meat begins to brown all over. Just before the meat is browned, add the soy sauce, capsicum, celery, mushrooms and shallots, stirring until the vegetables are tender.*
4. *Add the sesame seeds, Hoisin sauce, fish sauce and cooked noodles, and heat through.*

Variation – *If you don't like sesame seeds, crushed peanuts work well in this recipe. You can also add a tablespoon of peanut butter, and you have a healthy pad Thai.*

Asian vegetable stir fry with tofu (Serves 4 to 6)

1 teaspoon sesame oil
300g firm tofu, diced into bite-sized cubes
1 onion, chopped into small wedges
2 teaspoons crushed garlic
1 tablespoon light soy sauce
2 tablespoons oyster sauce
2 tablespoons water
1 red capsicum, seeded and chopped
½ cup baby carrots
1 cup snow peas
1 cup whole baby corn
1 cup shiitake mushrooms, sliced
¼ cup shallots, chopped
1 tablespoon pine nuts

1. *Add the oil and tofu to a non-stick pan on a medium heat, and stir fry gently until the tofu is cooked. Set aside.*

2. *Turn the heat up, and add the onion, garlic and a little water in the pan. Cook until the onion softens and the water evaporates.*

3. *Add the soy sauce, oyster sauce, water, capsicum, carrots, snow peas, baby corn, mushrooms and shallots, stirring until the vegetables are tender.*

4. *Return the cooked tofu to the dish and add the pine nuts, heating through.*

Hint – *If you can't find baby carrots, use carrot strips, and the baby corn can also be substituted with the canned variety. Just make sure they are well drained.*

Variation – *Other vegetables that would work well with this recipe include choy sum (Chinese broccoli), snake beans, zucchini, bean shoots and water chestnuts. If you don't like tofu, substitute chicken breast.*

Fat-burning power food – Soy products

Soy products such as tofu and soy milk are a good substitute or just an occasional alternative for animal products because they are a good source of protein. The regular consumption of soy products is also associated with a reduced risk of heart disease. Substituting plant protein products for animal-based protein foods can help to lower your saturated fat intake. It makes sense not to get all your protein from animal products all the time. Look for the low-fat versions of soy products such as milk and yoghurt to reduce your kilojoule intake.

 ## Fat-burning power food – Fish and seafood

Your health and your weight will benefit from eating fish and seafood regularly. The type of fat in fish and seafood (omega-3 fatty acid) can only be manufactured by your body in small amounts, so you need extra from your diet. All seafood contains varying amounts of omega-3 fatty acids, yet deep-sea fish tends to be the richest. Sardines, mackerel, salmon, rainbow trout, lake trout, herring, tuna and oysters are all good sources of omega-3 fatty acids.

 ## Fat-burning power food – Water-rich vegetables

Water rich vegetables have the lowest kilojoule content of virtually any food, and they are filling as well. Water-rich vegetables have 5 to 10 times fewer kilojoules than starchy vegetables such as potatoes, pumpkin and corn. Aim for 4 to 5 servings of water-rich vegetables each day, ideally as the foundation of your evening meal. This includes asparagus, celery, broccoli, zucchini, capsicum, cabbage, mushrooms, onions, tomato, green beans, spinach, leeks, eggplant, bok choy, baby corn and cucumber. Try to keep your starchy vegetable servings to around 1 to 2 per day.

Fish and seafood

(*RECIPE*)

Baked salmon and grilled vegetables (Serves 2)

½ Spanish onion, cut into wedges
1 red capsicum, cut into wide strips
2 small zucchini, quartered lengthways
2 roma tomatoes, quartered lengthways
2 long, narrow eggplants, quartered lengthways
2 teaspoons minced garlic
1 tablespoon mixed herbs
salt and pepper to taste
1 tablespoon olive oil
1 tablespoon lemon juice
1 tablespoon balsamic vinegar
2 Atlantic salmon fillets

1. *Preheat oven to 180°C.*

2. *In a small bowl, add the garlic, herbs, seasoning, oil, lemon juice and vinegar, and combine well.*

3. *Line a baking tray with baking paper, and add the onion, capsicum, zucchini, tomatoes and eggplant. Pour three quarters of the dressing over the vegetables, and mix them around, trying to cover them as evenly as possible.*

4. *Bake the vegetables in the oven for 15 minutes.*

5. *Remove the tray and toss around the vegetables, leaving a space for the fish. Depending on the size of your vegetables, some may be cooked at this stage, so remove any that are cooked to your liking.*

6. *Add the fish to the tray, and pour over the remaining dressing. Bake for a further 10 to 15 minutes, or until the fish is just cooked through.*

Hint – *Salmon is best when it's slightly pink in the centre. When overcooked, it gets dry and loses flavour.*

Variation – *Other vegetables you could bake include carrots, asparagus and thinly cut sweet potato. You could also top the fish with a tomato salsa, or a little low-fat mayonnaise.*

Fast feast dinner ideas

- **Steak and salad** – Grill a small, lean steak, and serve with a green salad dressed with balsamic vinegar and lemon juice.
- **Chicken pizza** – Spread a commercial wholemeal pizza base with tomato paste, and top with shredded chicken breast, capsicum, chopped tomato, red onion, mushrooms, pineapple, lean ham, and ricotta cheese.
- **Beef burger** – Using lean mince, egg whites and grated zucchini, make a hamburger patty. Grill and serve on a multigrain roll with salad vegetables.
- **Thai noodles with mussels** – Cook some low-fat two minute noodles. Steam some broccoli, capsicum and carrot. Combine noodles and vegetables with some mussels in brine (drained), oyster sauce and a few cashew nuts, and heat in a microwave.
- **Fast fried rice** – Heat a packet of three minute pre-cooked rice in the microwave. In a pan, heat some pre-cut vegetables, chopped ham, frozen peas and canned corn kernels. Add the heated rice and stir in some soy sauce for a fast fried rice.
- **Potato and tuna with salsa** – Cook a small potato with skin (pricked) in the microwave. Slice open the top, and spoon over some canned tuna, tomato salsa and cottage cheese. Heat the toppings and serve.
- **Warm salmon salad** – Bake a salmon fillet, and flake it over a salad made of baby spinach, almonds, cucumber, grated beetroot and ricotta cheese.
- **Cheese and chicken omelette** – Beat together one whole egg and an additional egg white. Add shredded chicken breast, chopped tomatoes, chopped onion, chopped fresh parsley and grated low-fat cheese. Serve with multigrain toast.

Snacks

Snacking is a good strategy as long as you are active, and that you stick to smaller portions during your main meals. While the oversupply of convenience foods has given snacking a bad reputation, well chosen snacks are helpful for weight loss. Healthy snacking can stabilise blood sugar levels and minimise the release of insulin, which can help you to lose weight and fat. By eating something every four hours, you can prevent the ravenous hunger and food cravings associated with low blood sugar levels. Try to snack on whole foods that are low in fat and sugars, and high in protein and/or fibre to fill you up and boost your energy levels.

Fruit

Like vegetables, fruit is packed with fibre and nutrients. But fruit is sweet because it's packed with sucrose, making it much higher in kilojoules than fibrous vegetables. Fruit is not an unhealthy food, and it's certainly a better snack that chocolate or biscuits. But it is high in kilojoules, so keep your portion sizes under control. Aim for about 2 daily servings of fruit as a snack or dessert (and 4–6 servings of vegetables). Berries are fat-burning power food because they are packed with nutrients, and they tend to be lower in kilojoules than most fruits.

(RECIPE)

Peach berry crumble (serves 1)

1 small ripe peach
¼ cup blueberries
1 teaspoon honey
1 pinch nutmeg
1 pinch ground cinnamon
1 tablespoon rolled oats
1 teaspoon desiccated coconut
2 tablespoons low-fat custard

1. *Preheat the oven to 180°C.*
2. *Remove the stone from the peach and cut the flesh into slices.*
3. *Put the sliced peach, blueberries, honey, nutmeg and cinnamon in an ovenproof bowl and mix together lightly.*
4. *Sprinkle the oats and then the coconut over the top.*
5. *Bake for 5 to 10 minutes, or until the topping goes slightly golden.*
6. *Pour the low-fat custard over the top.*

Hint – Canned peaches work just as well for this recipe.

Variation – Other fruits that could work well in this recipe include peeled apple, sultanas, pear, apricots, plums and stewed rhubarb. You could also use a small scoop of low-fat yoghurt or ice cream instead of the custard.

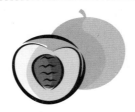

Trainer's notes – Plain fruit makes a great snack

See if you can identify 5 to 10 fruits that you could have as a snack, and try to keep them well stocked in your kitchen. Just some of the fruits you could choose include apples, banana, grapes, kiwifruit, strawberries, passion fruit, apricots, mandarins, oranges, mango, rockmelon, watermelon, peaches, plums, fruit salad, berries, nectarines, cherries, dates, figs, honeydew, paw paw (papaya), pears and pineapple.

RECIPE

Banana and walnut muffins (makes 8 to 12 muffins)

1 cup self-raising flour
½ cup wholemeal self-raising flour
¼ cup chopped walnuts or pecans
½ cup brown sugar
2 teaspoons cinnamon
2 ripe bananas, mashed
1 cup finely chopped dates
3 egg whites
½ cup low-fat vanilla yoghurt
1 teaspoon vanilla essence

1. Combine the self-raising flour, wholemeal self-raising flour, chopped nuts, brown sugar and cinnamon in a bowl and mix well.

2. In a separate bowl, mash the bananas, then add chopped dates, egg whites, yoghurt and vanilla essence and combine well.

3. Lightly stir the wet ingredients into the dry ingredients, and mix together as little as possible.

4. Spoon the mixture into lightly sprayed muffin tray, and bake at 180°C for 15 to 20 minutes, or until a skewer comes out clean.

Hint – These muffins look great with a little icing sugar sprinkled on top.

Variation – You could substitute grated carrot, stewed apple, blueberries or sultanas for the chopped dates in this recipe. You can also heat these and serve with a little low-fat ice cream or custard for a tasty dessert.

Yoghurt

Low-fat yoghurt makes a great snack, because it's high protein and calcium content makes it ideal for weight control. Yoghurt is also high in other vitamins and minerals such as B12 and magnesium, while its active cultures can help to balance your digestive system. Natural yoghurt is also very versatile, as it can be used to replace sour cream (mixed with a little lemon juice) or mayonnaise (mixed with a little mustard). Be wary of the sugar that comes with yoghurt. Combining plain low-fat yoghurt with fresh fruit and some nuts and seeds is the ideal choice, but you may have to dodge the rows of brightly coloured, sugar- and even jam-filled yoghurts that crowd the supermarket shelves. Artificially sweetened yoghurts are also OK in moderation. They are lower in kilojoules, but I am not a huge fan of sweeteners. Something that I do like, and which makes a great snack or dessert, is this yoghurt berry swirl delight.

(*RECIPE*)

Yoghurt-berry swirl delight (serves 1)

1 200g tub low-fat natural yoghurt
¼ cup berries, fresh or frozen
1 teaspoon maple syrup
1 tablespoon fresh berries

1. *Spoon the yoghurt into a dessert bowl or tall glass.*

2. *Put the berries and maple syrup in a blender or food processor and blend until smooth.*

3. *Swirl the berry syrup over the yoghurt, and top with fresh berries.*

 Fat-burning power food – Berries

Berries are top of the tree when it comes to health giving foods, including strawberries, raspberries, blackberries, and blueberries. They are packed with fibre, vitamins such as C and E, and are one of the richest sources of antioxidants. What's more, their bright colours make them look appetising, and they taste great. Eating them regularly has been shown to reduce the risk of cancer and heart disease. They are also strongly flavoured, so you can get the taste without too many kilojoules. They can be expensive, but try to have them whenever you can.

Dips

Dips are a very versatile food, and are very easy to prepare. They can last for several days in the fridge, so they can be on hand for a quick snack, entrée, as a filler or instead of butter on a sandwich, a pizza topping or a light meal. You can serve dips with cut vegetables such as capsicum, cucumber, celery, carrots, mushrooms, lettuce rolls or snow peas. They also work well with crusty wholemeal bread, dark rye bread, multigrain Cruskits and crackers, and toasted pita bread. Here are two of my favourites.

(*RECIPE*)

Eggplant dip (baba ghanoush) (makes 2 cups)

1 large eggplant
1 tablespoon tahini (sesame paste)
1 tablespoon olive oil
2 teaspoons minced or finely chopped garlic
1 tablespoon lemon juice
2 teaspoons sugar
1 teaspoon salt
1 teaspoon ground paprika
¼ cup chopped parsley

1. *Preheat oven to 220°C.*
2. *Line a baking tray with baking paper, and roast the eggplant for 30 to 40 minutes. The skin should blacken and blister, and the pulp should be soft.*
3. *Allow the eggplant to cool to room temperature, then peel and chop. Discard the skin.*
4. *Place in a blender or food processor the cooked eggplant, tahini, oil, garlic, lemon juice, sugar, salt, paprika and parsley. Blend until almost smooth. Refrigerate before serving.*

Hint – *The blacker the skin, the easier the eggplant will be to peel when it's cooled.*

Variation – *Other ingredients you can use in this recipe include black pepper, low-fat natural yoghurt, ground cumin and chilli sauce.*

Hummus (makes about 2 cups)

310g canned chickpeas, rinsed, drained
¼ cup water
1 tablespoon lemon juice
1 teaspoon minced garlic
1 tablespoon tahini (sesame paste)
1 teaspoon olive oil
1 teaspoon ground cumin
1 teaspoon paprika
½ teaspoon salt
pepper to taste

1. *Add the chickpeas, water, lemon juice and garlic to a food processor, and blend until smooth.*
2. *Add the tahini, oil, cumin, paprika, salt and pepper, and blend again.*
3. *Refrigerate before serving with pita bread, crackers or a salad.*

Hint – *Canned chickpeas are easy to use in this recipe, but you can also use the dried variety (soaked overnight).*

Variation – *Stir through 2 tablespoons of low-fat yoghurt for a creamier hummus.*

Fat-burning power food – Nuts and seeds

Nuts and seeds are high in fat and kilojoules, which has made them a dietary danger zone. But they are in fact rich in essential 'good' monounsaturated fats, and low in saturated fats, the type that raises your blood cholesterol levels. Because they also contain fibre and protein, nuts are effective at satisfying your appetite and preventing hunger. Just have a small serving, and avoid nuts that are roasted in oil or have added salt or sugar. This negates any health benefits associated with nuts. They are great in salads, stir fries, yoghurt and breakfast cereals, and are a good option for the occasional healthy snack. You can even make a spread for toast or cracker bread, like this recipe using pine nuts.

Pine nut spread

¼ cup sun-dried tomatoes (no oil)
2 tablespoons (30 g) pine nuts (lightly toasted)
1 cup basil, chopped
2 teaspoons minced garlic
1 teaspoon lemon juice
1 teaspoon sweet chilli sauce
1 teaspoon olive oil
salt and pepper to taste

1. *Soak the tomatoes in boiling water for 2 minutes, then drain.*

2. *Add the tomatoes, pine nuts, basil, garlic, lemon juice, sweet chilli sauce, oil and seasoning to a food processor, and blend into a paste.*

3. *Add a little water to get the desired consistency.*

Hint – *Use the semi-dried tomatoes that are literally dry. They are much lower in fat than the varieties soaked in oil. To toast pine nuts, just dry fry them in a pan on a low heat until they just begin to change colour. You can also stir through some additional whole pine nuts after the paste is blended if you prefer a chunkier spread.*

Variation – *This spread is also ideal as a dip with raw vegetables or low-fat crackers.*

You could also stir through a little white wine, and use it as a sauce with wholemeal pasta.

Trainer's notes – Get nuts about nuts

There are many varieties to choose from if you are looking to include small amounts of nuts and seeds in your diet. These include cashews, pecans, walnuts, pinenuts, pistachios, macadamias, hazelnuts, Brazil nuts, almonds, chestnuts, peanuts (although not officially a nut), pumpkin seeds, sunflower seeds and poppy seeds.

The versatile tomato

It's amazing what you can do with the humble tomato. You can use it as a base for salsa, as a dip or topping for baked fish. You can snack on sliced tomato on multigrain toast or cracker bread with cottage cheese and black pepper. But my favourite is bruschetta. It's a fantastic pre-dinner snack, or light lunch with a little green salad. I always like to have a batch of this recipe sitting in the fridge. Try it out for yourself.

--- (*RECIPE*)

Bruschetta (serves 4)

4 roma (plum) tomatoes, seeded and diced
½ red onion, finely chopped
2 cloves garlic, finely chopped
1 tablespoon balsamic vinegar
½ cup fresh basil, chopped
1 tablespoon extra virgin olive oil
1 teaspoon sugar
½ teaspoon salt
pepper to taste
1 multigrain bread stick, cut into discs approximately 1 cm thick

1. *Preheat oven to 200°C.*

2. *Combine the tomato, onion, garlic, vinegar, basil, oil, sugar, salt and pepper in a mixing bowl. Stir well and set aside.*

3. *Place the bread in the oven and toast until slightly golden, approximately 3 to 5 minutes.*

4. *Allow the bread to cool for a few minutes before topping with the tomato mixture.*

***Hint** – If you don't like the idea of raw onion and garlic, cook them off in a little water until the onion is transparent, and the water evaporates. To prevent the bread going soggy, serve the bread on a platter with the tomato mixture in a bowl so people can top the bread themselves.*

***Variation** – Where do I start? You can add chopped grilled capsicum, capers, chopped olives, anchovies, corn, avocado, feta cheese or slices of bocconcini cheese. Substitute the basil for coriander, and you have a salsa topping for fish or grilled vegetables. You can even add a little white wine, and use it as a sauce over wholemeal pasta. Finally, you can double the portions in this recipe, then boil the leftovers with a little water or stock, and blend it for a tasty tomato soup.*

Trainer's notes – Shopping list

With so many choices available at the supermarket, it's important that you are prepared and organised when you go food shopping. After all, if you don't buy junk at the supermarket, there's less likely to be any around, and you are less likely to eat it. You probably have heard the tip to always shop on a full stomach, and that advice holds true. You will be less inclined to buy treats. But more importantly, shop with a list that caters for all the foods in your meal plans. Try to make sure the 10 fat-burning power foods appear regularly on your shopping list.

Fast feast snack ideas

- fresh fruit salad
- low-fat muesli bars
- pretzels
- canned tuna (in brine) with tomato on multigrain cracker bread
- vegetable-based soups
- breakfast cereal and skim milk
- baked beans on toast
- rice cakes with ham, tomato, cottage cheese and pepper
- coloured rice crackers
- air-popped popcorn
- multigrain English muffins with marmalade
- wholemeal crumpets and creamed honey
- raisin toast with jam
- tomato salsa and vegetable sticks
- lite cup-a-soups
- low-fat cottage cheese and pineapple on toast
- low-fat custard and canned fruit
- sorbet
- UP & GO breakfast drinks (or other pre-made smoothies)
- flavoured bread sticks
- small portions of dried fruits with nuts and seeds

9

Training for advanced walkers

IT'S TIME to step up your walking program. Faster walking means faster results. If you feel ready to start with the advanced walking program, or have just completed the 8-week Walk Off Weight program, read on about how you can take your walking routine to a new level.

Heart rate training

Choosing the right balance between frequency, intensity, type and duration of exercise will determine the level of fat loss or fitness you achieve. While frequency, duration and type are easy to record, the most accurate way to measure your intensity is with your heart rate. You can achieve different goals by working at different levels or percentages of your maximum heart rate (MHR). MHR is determined by subtracting your age from 220. By training at different levels or percentages of your MHR, you can achieve different health and fitness goals. If you are a beginner, work at around 50% to 65% of MHR. This level is also good for long duration walks (40 to 60 minutes). As your fitness improves and exercise gets easier, it's best to train at 65% to 85% of your MHR. This range is ideal for fat burning, and will also help to boost your aerobic fitness. The chart below is a guide to maximum heart rate and training zones for different ages. You can apply this information by taking your pulse, but a heart rate monitor makes it simple.

Age	Fat burning for beginners 50%–65%	Advanced fat burning 65%–85%	MHR
20	100–130	130–170	200
25	98–127	127–166	195
30	95–124	124–162	190
35	93–120	120–157	185
40	90–117	117–153	180
45	88–114	114–149	175
50	85–111	111–145	170
55	83–107	107–140	165
60	80–104	104–136	160
65	78–101	101–132	155

Interval training for walkers

Interval training offers a change from steady state exercise, where you always work at the same level. It involves the use of short bursts (around 30 to 60 seconds) of intense effort followed by a recovery period that is mixed into your normal exercise routine. This higher level of intensity really boosts the kilojoule-burning effect of your exercise, and adds an extra dimension to your training. Using short bursts to work harder than normal helps your body adapt to a higher level of fitness and stamina, and take you to a level that steady state exercise can not. It allows you to train at a much higher level, but in small, tolerable doses. To give you a better idea what interval training is, I have included a sample workout below.

- 5 minutes – slow walk warm up
- 1 minute – walk as fast as you can
- 30 seconds – catch your breath
- repeat 8 times
- walk at a moderate pace to a steep hill or a long flight of stairs
- walk as fast as you can up the hill/stairs
- walk slowly down and catch your breath
- repeat 4 times
- walk at a moderate pace until you are fairly close to home
- 3 minutes – walk slowly to cool down

Science says – Women less likely to push themselves

A recent survey found that women are less likely than men to engage in vigorous exercise. These results could have serious implications for women, who already find it harder than men to lose weight and fat. Interval training is an ideal way for women to integrate more vigorous exercise into their routine.

Intervals help you overcome a plateau

As you lose weight, and get fitter, you will gradually burn fewer kilojoules from walking. After all, there is less of you to carry around. Unless you continue to push the envelope, increase your intensity and exert yourself at a higher level, your results will get harder to come by. This is why people often experience a plateau, where they have a long period without much change in weight or body shape. As I've already discussed in Chapter 3, the majority of walkers don't get all the benefits they could out of walking because they don't push themselves. Don't rely exclusively on interval training, as it is too strenuous and taxing on your body. But interval training is a great complement to your walking routine two or three times a week.

Does interval training help with weight loss?

When you want to lose weight and fat, the key is to burn off as many kilojoules as you can. Interval training allows you to burn kilojoules at a higher rate for a longer period of time, because you get the chance to recover. This stronger level of effort will also push your body towards a higher level of fitness and fat burning. If you find it hard to make the time to exercise, intervals help you achieve more with less. Other advantages for fat loss include a bigger boost in your metabolic rate and a greater reduction in your appetite.

Advantages of interval training

- Bigger boost of your metabolic rate
- Increased kilojoule use
- Higher level of aerobic fitness
- Higher level of weight and fat loss
- Helps you break through a weight-loss plateau
- Increased appetite suppression
- Increase in energy levels
- Prevention of boredom
- Better training for sports

Trainer's tip – Go on, challenge yourself

If you have been exercising at the same level for some time now, why not challenge yourself, and do something a little different? Next time you are out walking, try some intervals. Walking is a low-intensity activity, so you really need to go fast, swing your arms vigorously and push yourself. At the end of a hard interval, you should feel really puffed, and feel like you need the rest interval. You will burn more kilojoules in the same amount of time, and increase your chances of getting results. What have you got to lose?

WARNING – If you are very overweight, or have a history of heart disease, don't push yourself too hard. Make your intervals only slightly harder than normal. Check with your doctor if you have any concerns.

Cross training for walkers

Cross training is an exercise strategy where you incorporate a variety of different activities into your routine. By supplementing your primary exercise (walking) with different activities, you can combine the benefits of different exercises to achieve a common goal. It can help to strengthen muscles not used during walking, and spare muscles that are used during walking from overuse and injury. An example of a cross-training program designed to lose weight and body fat is tabled below.

Day	Physical activity	Planned duration	Actual duration
Monday	Fast walk	40 minutes	
Tuesday	Cycling	60 minutes	
Wednesday	Lift weights (25) Very fast walk (15)	40 minutes total	
Thursday	Soccer	120 minutes	
Friday	Fast walk	40 minutes	
Saturday	Lift weights (25) Very fast walk (15)	40 minutes total	
Sunday	Gentle beach walk	60 minutes	

But isn't walking the best way to burn fat?

I can't speak highly enough of the benefits of walking as a fat-loss exercise, and the role it can play in helping you lose weight and fat. One simple way to cross train is to incorporate different styles of walking, such as those outlined in Chapter 2. But once your initial 8-week challenge is over, combining different activities with walking can make your exercise routine more interesting, challenging and fun. Some of these different activities also offer unique fat-loss benefits that walking simply can't match. Walking is such a low-intensity exercise that you may need additional activities to take your workouts and your body to another level. Because I want you to get results, I'd like you to learn more about these activities, and consider adding them to your routine.

Will cross training help me lose more weight and fat?

Cross training is ideal for fat loss, and can also benefit your heart health and cardiovascular fitness. If you've completed the 8-week challenge, and want to add something different to your program, cross training is ideal. A major benefit from the extra variety is the boost to your motivation, especially if you get bored doing the same thing every day. Adding variety and mixing things up is like a breath of fresh air to your exercise routine. By performing different cardiovascular activities that you enjoy, you will be more likely to incorporate them into daily life, and stick with exercise over the long term. Once your walking program is well established, there are a variety of additional activities you can choose from. The following activities can be a great addition to your routine, and have been highlighted due to their additional fat-loss benefits.

Running, and run/walks

Yes, I know this is a book about walking. But this chapter is about adding variety to your walking routine. If the thought of 'running' doesn't make you cringe, it's something you should consider. The debate on whether you should walk or run depends upon your weight and level of fitness. If you are walking fast for over an hour without much duress, running has some advantages in terms of weight loss and fitness training. The extra intensity can add some real impact to your workouts. You don't have to run the whole way, but include short runs during your walk. However, if you weigh over 100 kilograms, only run: if you are very fit; are without any existing knee problems; can do so on grass or sand; and are wearing shoes with excellent cushioning. Otherwise, it's too stressful on your joints.

The advantages of running over walking

- Running burns 3 times more kilojoules than walking.
- Running has a bigger impact on boosting your metabolism.
- You get a better workout in less time.
- Running gives you a quicker path to fat and weight loss.
- If you can walk fast, you should be able to run.
- Little bursts of running add intensity to your walks.
- You are more likely to get a 'runner's high'.

 ### Science says – Running versus walking

A recent study comparing the weight-loss effects of running and walking found that, for people who hadn't exercised in a number of years, it didn't matter what they did. Both the runners and walkers lost weight, although the runners did lose slightly more. It seems running is a better option for advanced walkers, not beginners.

Cycling

Do you have a bicycle sitting idle in the garage, or a stationary bike collecting dust? Cycling is one of the most effective all-round exercises for aerobic conditioning and fat burning. Cycling burns kilojoules while strengthening and toning the muscles in your legs and butt without impact. Sitting on the seat while pedalling will predominantly use your hip and thigh muscles, while standing and pedalling uses the buttocks and calf muscles. Do both for variety and balance. To focus on weight and fat loss, select an easy gear (or low resistance on an exercise bike) and aim for a fast pedalling speed (90 to 100 revolutions per minute). Cycling can add variety to your routine, and allows you to see so much more during your workouts. The fresh air in your face and the rhythm you get into can give you a real buzz. Mountain biking is also popular, and while a little more extreme, is one of the most enjoyable ways to burn off kilojoules. Exercise bikes give you a smoother, more consistent ride, and are a good option on miserable days. You can also buy a device called a 'trainer' that supports the back wheel of your bicycle and allows you to use it indoors. This is like having the best of both worlds. Because cycling is not weight bearing (the seat supports your weight), aim for longer sessions of exercise to maximise kilojoule use and fat burning.

Strength training

Walkers can benefit from lifting weights to boost fat loss and strengthen the upper body, which is used very little during walking. Strength training can also be referred to as weight training or resistance training, but it all means the same thing. It involves moving your body against a resistance, such as dumbbells, barbells, weight machines or your own body weight. Strength training helps to combat the effects of inactivity and ageing, and offers a wide range of benefits, including muscle toning, increased bone density, improved posture, improved blood sugar control and reduced risk of heart disease.

Can lifting weights help with weight loss?

We all gradually lose muscle tissue as we get older, starting from the age of twenty. Because this slows down your metabolic rate, the speed at which your body burns off kilojoules, ageing often results in fat storage. This effect is sometimes called middle-aged spread. Lifting weights can reverse this process, helping to protect and strengthen your muscles, and boost your metabolic rate to help burn fat. Lifting weights a few times a week helps to activate your muscle tissue like no other exercise, and counteract the effects of ageing. Muscle burns more kilojoules than any other body tissue, so it makes sense to use it, strengthen it and tone it.

Trainer's tip – Weights won't make you bulky

Don't worry about getting big muscles from lifting weights. That's one of the greatest health and fitness myths known to man. Males have the potential to bulk up if they dedicate their lives to it, take supplements and lift extremely heavy weights. But that's not the type of lifting I am encouraging you to do. Of the thousands of women I have trained and seen trained based on the guidelines mentioned in this chapter, none have bulked up. But they can dramatically improve their strength, muscle tone and energy levels.

Ball games and team sports

There are a variety of activities out there for every level of fitness and sporting ability, including volleyball, basketball, soccer, touch football, and tennis. Team sports are an intermittent activity, where you stop and start regularly, so they are not as good for fat loss as continuous activities like walking, running, cycling, and paddling. They still give you the opportunity to improve aerobic fitness, improve strength and burn significant amounts of kilojoules. But they offer you much more in other areas, such as fun, teamwork, social interaction and learning new skills. You tend to develop an unwavering commitment to the team, which is great for your motivation. This can also create an environment where you push yourself harder than normal so you don't let the side down. To get the most benefits, try to be an active player and get involved as much as you can. These types of activities add real variety to your routine, and in some ways you won't even feel like you're exercising. But there is a higher risk of injury due to the short burst of exertion placing extra demands on your muscles, ligaments and joints. So warm up properly, strengthen the appropriate muscle for your chosen activity, and stretch after the game.

Paddling

Paddling a boat is a great form of low impact cross training for walkers, because your lower body gets a break while your upper body helps to burn kilojoules and fat. In addition to working your arms, the twisting and balancing also targets your abdominals, buttocks and core strength. You could try a kayak, a canoe, a wave ski or even dragon boating. If you don't mind the thought of facing backwards as you go forwards, rowing is another option if you have access to a boat. It's a great way to get outdoors, see some of the nicer parts of your local waterways, and get away from it all. Why not give it a try by seeking out a local club or hire centre. If you are a little hesitant, go with a friend and try out a 2-person canoe before taking on the challenge of a 1-person kayak. Like all activities, you can perform intervals, with short bursts of power and speed paddling mixed in with longer-duration, gentler movement. As your upper body strength and fitness develops, you might eventually want a craft of your own. If you are a beginner, or if you really want to take your paddling to another level, it will help to get a lesson to perfect your technique.

Gym membership

Joining a fitness centre has some advantages if you feel comfortable in that environment, and you take steps to get the most out of your membership. Gyms can be a good supplement to your walking routine, especially on cold, wet windy days, or if you don't have room for exercise equipment of your own. Most gyms offer a large variety of cardiovascular-based exercise machines and strength-training equipment, with a choice of exercise classes to suit most age groups and fitness levels. If the classes appeal to you, make sure you feel comfortable and coordinated, and choose classes that keep your heart rate up so you burn kilojoules and fat. Alternatively, you might want to try boxing, Pilates, yoga or stretching classes to add variety. When choosing cardiovascular equipment, treadmills mimic the action of walking or running, so they are ideal for fat burning. Steppers, rowers, elliptical trainers and exercise bikes all keep your heart rate up if you push yourself hard enough, and will give you an effective fat-burning workout. If you want to add resistance training to your routine, the wide array of dumbbells, barbells and weight-training machines at a gym will be almost impossible to match in the home environment. Just make sure to begin gradually, and seek out expert help if you are unsure about the correct weight or technique. A final consideration is to try before you buy. Go for a casual visit to see if you feel comfortable before signing a contract or committing yourself financially.

Things to weigh up when joining a gym

- Is the gym a well-established business?
- Is the location easy for you?
- Are the staff friendly and helpful?
- Do they have a good selection of the equipment you want to use?
- Is the gym packed out at the main times you want to attend?
- Is the equipment clean and well maintained?
- Does the gym have lockers for your valuables?
- Is there childcare available?
- Is there plenty of parking?
- Can you put your membership on hold?

Personal training

Once thought to be the realm of celebrities and supermodels, personal trainers are gaining popularity with the wider community. Personal trainers give you individual attention, and structure exercise programs around your specific needs. This not only increases the safety of your exercise program, but also increases your likelihood of getting results. An appointment with a personal trainer adds to your commitment to exercise, and can really help encourage and motivate you. As an addition to your walking program, try to do activities with a trainer that you can't do yourself. This might include strength training, boxing, using different exercise equipment or simply walking at a higher level than you would push yourself. This can be especially helpful when you are just learning a new activity such as strength training. Prices vary dramatically depending on the duration of your session, the quality of the trainer, if you are prepared to share your session, how many sessions you do a week, and how many sessions you pay for in advance.

Things to weigh up when hiring a personal trainer

- How many days a week/month do you want to be trained?
- What qualifications and training does the trainer have?
- Is the trainer currently registered with a fitness industry association?
- How experienced is the trainer?
- Does the trainer specialise in a particular area (pregnancy, weights, fat loss)?
- Where does the training take place (home, gym, studio, outdoors)?
- Does the trainer have first aid qualifications and insurance in case a client is injured?
- Can the trainer fit you into their schedule at a time that suits you?
- What is the trainer's cancellation policy?

Other popular cross-training activities

- swimming
- surfing/body boarding
- roller blading (inline skating)
- elliptical trainer (exercise machine)
- stepper (exercise machine)
- aerobic videos or exercise classes on television
- dancing
- boxing for fitness

10

Get motivated

'Go the extra mile. It's less crowded'. – Author unknown

10 ways to get started, and stick with it

A lot of people start exercise programs with great gusto, only to find their walking shoes collecting dust within a month or two. When you first make the decision to change, you generally don't have to worry about motivation, because it comes naturally. But when your initial enthusiasm dies down, it's important to have some strategies to call upon that can help keep you moving and motivated. There will be days when you don't feel like it, but the following tips will help to maintain your interest and keep you moving.

1 – Have something to strive for

That's what this book is all about – striving to lose weight and fat. Just how much that goal means to you will ultimately determine your level of results. Long-term goals are vital to your success because they provide direction, motivation and focus. Achieving these types of goals is a reward in itself. Try to think about (or better still write down) why you want to lose weight. How is excess body fat holding you back? How would your life improve if you were leaner and healthier? What scares you the most about staying the same? Keep your answers to these questions close by, and call on them whenever you are experiencing a motivational down turn. Goal setting might seem a bit of a waste of time, but it only takes a few minutes, and it can really help to give you direction and focus. Beyond your weight- and fat-loss goals, you can also set some goals based on your walking. You could try to beat your personal best time or distance over a set walk, or train for an event like a fun run. These personal challenges can be one of most effective ways to motivate yourself.

Examples of long-term goals

- Walk a marathon
- Walk in a local fun run
- Walk between two towns or suburbs

- Walk the Milford Sound in New Zealand
- Walk the Kokoda Track in Papua New Guinea
- Walk the Inca trails
- Walk around Uluru
- Walk a stretch of beaches
- Walk 7 kilometres in an hour
- Walk a challenging distance or duration

2 – Have a plan

Setting a weight loss goal is what's called an outcome- or results-based goal. This is the destination that you seek. But how do you get there? That's where short-term process goals come into play, and are like stepping stones to help you reach your destination. Process goals are the specific actions, steps, behaviours, skills, moods and thinking processes you will need for your outcome to eventuate. You have much more control over the process than you do over the results. Keeping a food diary or an activity journal can help you put the pieces together. Write it down and create a timeline, breaking your goal down into specific, measurable pieces. By focusing on completing the 8-week walking program in this book, you have a ready-made process goal. By following the 8-week challenge, you have an action plan to help you complete the process. After completing the 8-week walking challenge, I would strongly encourage you to set some new goals. You can copy the format I have used and create your own action plans to help you achieve them.

Examples of process goals

- Walk for 5 days each week for the next month
- Plan my meals for the next seven days
- Drink water before eating breakfast, lunch and dinner
- Have 3 alcohol-free nights each week
- Use my dumbbells twice a week
- Save $5 a week for a new pair of walking shoes
- Add interval training to my walks once a week
- Go for a 3-hour walk once a month

3 – Act on your plan

Talk, words, thoughts, goals, plans and intentions are all important, but somewhere in there, you need to take action. You need to put your plans into practice. Make it a priority and make the time by making an appointment. Schedule your walks just as you would schedule other important tasks. Plan your exercise sessions in advance and record them in your diary. Lack of time is less of a problem if you organise your time well. Allocate a time that best suits your schedule, be it morning, noon or night. Have indoor options for miserable days, such as some cross training, or a casual visit at your local gym. By getting organised, you are helping to follow through with your plan and committing yourself to a course of action. Once that course of action is started, success breeds success, and you can begin to generate some momentum. Habits are developed through consistency and regular practice.

Tips on how to fit walking into a busy schedule

- Watch less television
- Get a treadmill, and walk while you watch television
- Walk in your lunch break
- If you only have limited time to exercise, walk faster
- Incorporate walking into everyday life (incidental walking)
- Walk in the morning, when there are less unscheduled appointments
- Have a walking meeting/social catch up
- Minimise your travel time to and from exercise
- Prepare your shoes and clothes the night before

4 – Revel in the change and the challenge

Doing more walking, and changing the way you eat is not easy, but the results are well worth it. Change is stressful, but an open mind and self-belief can make all the difference. There is every reason to think that this time will be successful if you follow my plan. If you want to change your body shape, improve your health and lose weight, you'll have to change your lifestyle. Increasing the quantity of kilojoules you burn through physical activity is one of the cornerstones of success. What a great opportunity to try something new, and make health and fitness more of a priority than you did before. You may have to give up some of your old habits, but there's no time like the present. Don't put your life and your health on hold while wasting time on things that aren't necessary or good for you. The time you invest in walking and eating more healthily will pay you back 5-fold by giving you more energy, increasing the quality of your sleep, and reducing your risk of suffering several diseases. At times, these changes will be difficult – expect them to be, but it's these very changes that increase your chances of getting well, and getting results. As you progress towards getting the results you seek, and achieving what you set out to do, you may find your goals and priorities shifting. As you continue to make changes, regularly revisit your goals, especially if your new level of fitness requires a more demanding challenge.

5 – Use the buddy system

Making changes and sticking to them is always easier with company. See if you can find a friend, family member or partner who enjoys walking, and schedule a few workouts together each week. While you should be able to hear your breath while you walk, you can still carry on a conversation. It certainly beats catching up over coffee and cake. Having a training partner gives you an outside source of motivation, encouraging and supporting you, and making your walks more enjoyable. Having someone else to depend on, and who depends on you, makes it harder to skip a workout. Try to find someone with the same goals and a similar level of fitness to you. An equally fit training partner will challenge you to keep up the pace on days when you are a little off, while you can push them if they are slacking.

6 – Walk the dog

Dogs can make excellent training partners, and serve as a great source of motivation to keep you walking regularly. The size of your dog will determine how fast and therefore how effective your walks are. Larger dogs will walk faster, but even small dogs can add some variety to your routine. Dogs demand regular exercise, and this will have health benefits for both of you. If you only share a walk together on weekends, don't push your dog too hard. Remember to keep both of you well hydrated. Don't forget to take a lead and a plastic bag, and be aware of providing a comfortable space between your dog and other walkers. If your dog constantly stops to sniff things, or offer something for other dogs to sniff, go for a longer walk to get the maximum benefits. If your dog is well trained, try to keep up a good, steady pace, and enjoy walking with your best friend. If you don't have a dog, see if you can join a friend who does, or offer to walk their dog for them.

Why dogs are good training partners

- They need to be walked every day
- They make you feel guilty if they don't walk
- They can behave badly if they don't get walked
- They are ready to go when you are
- They never have an excuse not to exercise

- They provide added safety during your walks
- They don't slow down for hills
- They can vary their speed to suit you
- You will probably wear out before they do

Science says – The rewards of pet ownership

Research suggests that there is a link between pet ownership and better health. Pet ownership was shown to lower blood pressure, prolong life and increase the likelihood of regular exercise.

7 – Get real about your results

It's important that the things you strive for and the goals you set yourself are achievable. If you expect quick results, you can expect a quick disappointment. It's better to have realistic expectations, and focus on the long term. There's not much point starting something if you're not going to continue. The lifestyle you lead to get results has to be maintained if you want those results to last. You should expect a slow adaptation to gradual lifestyle changes. You should also expect there to be periods of time where there are no noticeable changes in your body shape. The body will shed weight in a step-like pattern, not in a continuous fashion. These plateaus should happen, and are a normal part of the process. As you get fitter, you will need to increase the intensity of your walks to continue to improve, and break through a plateau. This is not to discourage you. In fact, by acknowledging these well-known facts, you will avoid disappointment, and prevent a motivational shut down.

8 – Have the occasional easy day

There are always going to be days when you are tired, you don't feel like going, and there seem to be a mountain of excuses piling up. The old you would have stayed in bed, but you have committed to walking, and this is your chance to step out of your shell. Why not go anyway – but take it really easy. Just go for a stroll. You can forget about posture, pace and personal bests. Mentally, it just takes the pressure right off you, knowing you can just relax and enjoy the sights, but still be out there doing something. Yeah, sure – it's better to go for 40 minutes, but 15 minutes is still worth it, and can keep you from feeling like you've failed. Easy days are also helpful if you are a little sore, which can happen when you are just beginning your 8-week program.

9 - Bounce back from setbacks

By managing your health and your energy levels, you are much more likely stay on top of things. It's going to be a lot easier to get yourself up for a walk after a good night's sleep rather than after a late night and a few too many gin and tonics. It's also important for you to face up to the obstacles that can block your momentum. Challenges and setbacks are a part of life, and the reality is you will face some along the way. But it's how you bounce back from these obstacles that can make a world of difference. Learn to anticipate them, expect them, prepare for them, and don't give up if things go astray. If you let things slip, think about how you could respond next time if a similar circumstance arose. Learn from it and move on. Testing times are just another challenge that help determine your true level of commitment. Don't use it as an excuse to undo all your good work. Adjust your plans, don't abandon them.

Common setbacks to prepare yourself for

- Family commitments and stress
- Holidays and special occasions
- Procrastination and excuse making
- The desire to focus on your results instead of the process
- Lack of time through work or social commitments
- Changes to your body shape that are slower than expected
- Plateaus, or periods of no noticeable change in your body shape
- Craving foods or drinks you have cut back on
- Friends wanting you to indulge in treats to ease their guilt

10 - Make it fun

For exercise to become a lifelong habit, it's important that you enjoy it. Fun means different things to different people, but a little bit of creativity and a fun attitude can help to make walking more pleasurable for anyone. Consider the exercise variables that will determine how much you enjoy your walks, such as the importance you place on social contact, location (indoors or outdoors), intensity and competitiveness. Think about your own personality, your likes and turn offs, and look for ways you can add interest. What aspects of your last exercise program did you enjoy, and what made you quit? By generating enthusiasm and creating an environment where you look forward to your walks, you will be more likely to stick with it. One great way to enjoy your walks is to listen to music, talkback radio or even talking books on a portable device. The distraction will help you to exercise for longer, and make your workouts feel shorter. It may also help to think about the aspects of exercise that you don't like, and eliminate them. For example, if you hate walking in the cold, you could consider hiring a treadmill over winter.

Ways to add fun to your walks

- Change your scenery regularly
- Join a walking group for social interaction
- Change your walking surface regularly
- Listen to your favourite music
- Have a recorded time to beat over a set distance
- Use your walks as creative thinking time
- Enter a race or fun run
- Use rewards (not food) when you overcome a challenge
- Have a session with a personal trainer
- Add interval training to your walks

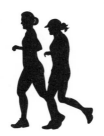

11

Treadmills

Treadmills – the king of exercise machines

Treadmills are one of the most popular forms of exercise equipment, and are a great way to make sure you stick to your walking routine. They are ideal if personal safety, allergies or bad weather limit your outdoor walking, or if you like to exercise in front of the television. They are also a good choice of exercise equipment if you are visiting a gym. While not quite as good as walking outside for your balance, they make up for it by giving you a consistent speed, helping you develop a good rhythm. Treadmills allow you to monitor the precise speed and incline of your walks, which is an excellent way to measure your progress, and see your improvements over time. A number of models even provide cushioning, where the deck absorbs your weight to reduce the impact on your knees and ankles. Follow these helpful tips when choosing and using your treadmill to maximise the effectiveness of your workout.

Science says – Treadmills versus road running

A recent study showed that running on a treadmill instead of running on hard surfaces reduces your chances of a developing a stress fracture of the lower leg by 48 per cent.

Starting out on a treadmill

Before you hop on a treadmill, stand beside it and familiarise yourself with the electronic display. Make sure you know how to raise and lower the speed and incline, and get a good feel for the controls. Identify where the stop or emergency stop button is, just in case you ever feel dizzy or faint (although it is best not to stop suddenly). When you feel ready to start walking, grab the handles, and stand with your feet on the foot rails (usually either side of the belt). Start the machine at low incline (1 to 2%) and a very slow speed of around 2 to 3 kilometres per hour (1 to 2 miles). Keeping your hands on the handrails, and your weight on one foot, 'paw' the moving belt a few times with the other foot. This will help you to get a better feel for the speed the treadmill is travelling at, and allows you to lower it if you have any concerns.

Getting on board for the first time

You are now ready to step onto the moving belt and start walking. When you get on, take long steps, look straight ahead and stand tall. Avoid looking down, or trying to push the belt with your feet as you hold on with your hands. Normally when you walk, the scenery moves around you, and you feel a light breeze. On a treadmill, this doesn't happen, and it can be a little disorientating at first. This is normal, so give yourself a little time to adjust. When you feel comfortable, slowly increase the speed to 4 to 6 km/hr (3 to 4 mph), and stay at that speed for a few minutes. If you are feeling really comfortable, let go of one handle and swing your arm in tune with the opposite leg. Do this for a minute or two, and then swap swinging arms. It may feel a little uncomfortable, but you just need to try and walk as naturally as possible.

Trainer's tip – Position your treadmill carefully

Position your treadmill so that the end of the belt is at least 1 to 2 metres away from any walls, windows or furniture. That way, in the unlikely case that you get thrown off, you won't hit anything and injure yourself. It's also important to be aware that when you are just starting out, people have a tendency to veer in the direction they are looking. This can be dangerous if your foot goes off the belt. If you are going to watch TV while using your treadmill, try to position it directly in front of the treadmill to prevent any potential problems.

When to let go of the handles

Practise holding on with only one hand until you are ready to walk hands free. This could take several attempts, but practise until you feel comfortable. Walking on a treadmill is no substitute for walking outside if you hold onto the handles. If you are still learning, or feel much more comfortable digging your claws in to the handles, fair enough. But this is also the best time for you to learn good habits. Holding onto the handrails alters your body's natural walking mechanics, and is not ideal for your knees or back. Swinging your arms will also maximise the fat-burning effect of using a treadmill. You will burn more kilojoules walking at a slower speed and swinging your arms than walking at a faster speed and hanging on. Use the same technique that I outlined in Chapter 2, where you bend your arms at a 90 degree angle.

Times when it's okay to use the treadmill handrails

- You are an absolute beginner
- You are just getting on to a moving belt
- You want to adjust the settings
- You are rapidly slowing down the speed
- You are rapidly lowering the incline
- You need to turn around to talk to somebody
- You want to check your heart rate
- You are about to fall off the back
- You feel faint, dizzy or nauseous or experience chest pain
- You want to get off

What's the right speed?

The right speed for you on a treadmill will depend on your incline, your level of fitness, your leg length, your level of comfort and experience, the duration of your walk, and how hard you are prepared to push yourself. Start off at a steady pace where you feel comfortable, and build it up to a challenging speed where you still feel safe. You might need to adjust the speed slightly if you are doing shorter (less than 10 minutes) or longer (longer than 40 minutes) walks. As you get used to your treadmill, walking speed will become a no-brainer, as you will set the speed at the same level you did previously. When you find this speed a little easy, you can up the ante slightly. This is the beauty of treadmills, where you can constantly strive to beat your personal best speed, distance or duration.

Trainer's tip – Find the right speed for you

The ideal walking speed for maximal kilojoule use is at a pace where you feel like you could break into a run, but you continue to walk. This is an inefficient movement, and it burns lots of kilojoules since you fight your body's natural tendency to jog.

What's the right incline?

The incline on a treadmill has a dramatic influence over the kilojoules you burn during your workouts. Start off on 2 per cent, which is equivalent to a flat walk. This is your benchmark, and I advise you never to go below this level unless you have calf pain or shin splints. As you get fitter, a higher gradient will challenge you, and help you burn significantly more kilojoules and fat. The incline on a treadmill is a great feature, and an absolute blessing for walkers. It allows you to burn kilojoules at a rate similar to running, but without the jarring and stress on your joints. Once your walking speed gets to point where you don't feel like you can go any faster, pump up the incline to re-invigorate your training, and your fat burning.

Science says – Increase the incline slightly

A recent study compared the kilojoules used on a treadmill with the kilojoules used during a normal walk outdoors at an equivalent speed. It was found that the treadmill needs to be set at a gradient of 2 per cent for it to be equal with the kilojoules used during a normal flat walk. This is because there is less air resistance. No difference was found between a treadmill and walking outdoors at slower speeds, but as speed increased, so did the difference in kilojoule use.

Key points about using your treadmill effectively

- Keep the gradient at a minimum of 2 per cent to match the effects of walking on a flat surface.
- Unless you are just starting out, don't hang onto the handles.
- Use the various programs and patterns on your treadmill to add variety, challenge yourself and prevent boredom.
- Cool down by walking at a slower speed after your workout. Don't stop cold.
- Before you use a treadmill, familiarise yourself with the electronic display. Learn how to adjust the speed and incline settings, and locate the stop button.

Treadmill workouts

If your treadmill has a number of different programs, try them all, and find a couple you enjoy. It helps to be familiar with all your options if you want to get the most out of your treadmill, and yourself. Programs can add variety if you get a little bored doing the same thing all the time. Once you have recorded some of the times and distances you have achieved, you then have something to beat next time. That then becomes the ideal program for you, a program where you try to beat your personal best. It's the one that you do for a little longer than last time, or a little faster, or a little steeper, or that takes you a little further. That's how you burn fat and get fit – gradually and progressively. That way, you get the most out of your treadmill, and help prevent it from becoming an expensive dust collector.

Science says – Don't hang on

A study investigating the use of your arms on a treadmill showed that you can burn over 30 per cent more kilojoules by swinging your arms. Kilojoule use jumped from around 40 kilojoules per minute up to 60 kilojoules per minute by swinging the arms vigorously.

Five fun treadmill routines

Workout	Speed	Incline	Duration	Variations/ Comments
Beginner	5 km/h (3 mph)	2 %	20 minutes	If you find the speed easy, up the incline for the last 15 minutes.
Walk Off Weight	6.5 to 7.4 km/h (4 to 4.5 mph)	3 %	35 minutes	For an extra challenge, walk at a faster speed for the first 30 seconds of each minute for 10 of the 35 minutes.
Advanced	7.5 to 8 km/h (4.5 to 5 mph)	4 %	30 minutes	For an extra challenge, up the incline for the last 15 minutes.
Interval session	6 km/h warm up, 10 km/h intervals and 4 km/h rests.	3 %	3-minute warm up, 1-minute intervals and 1-minute rests. Repeat 8 to 10 times	Use the same speed, and vary the incline. You can also alter the duration of the interval and rest periods for a different workout.
Treadmill and weights on the side	6.5 km/h	2 %	3-minute warm up, 2-minute intervals and weights exercises in between. Repeat 6 to 8 times	If you don't have weights for the strength-training exercises, use body weight exercises such as push ups, sit ups, dips, lunges, squats and calf raises.

Choosing a treadmill

Research has shown that a treadmill is the most used piece of exercise equipment. Even so, there are some important variables you will need to weigh up before buying or renting a treadmill. While they are great machines for weight control and fat loss, it pays to do your homework. Treadmills have many features and specifications, so it's important to weigh up which ones are most important to you. The following table outlines the most important features you will need to consider. It's an investment in your future health and wellness, so don't rush in until you know what you want.

Feature	Considerations
Power	The power of a treadmill motor is usually rated in horsepower. The power of the motor will reflect the amount of weight a treadmill can comfortably carry, so check which models are suitable for you. A larger, more powerful motor will run more effectively and last longer than a smaller one.
Incline	The incline on a treadmill can be altered either electronically or manually. Manual treadmills cannot have their incline changed while in motion, which is very inconvenient. Electronic incline can range from 5 to 20 per cent on some models, although it will increase your costs. Electronic incline is a great way to add variety and intensity to your walks, and well worth the extra expense.
Speed	Some treadmills are branded as walkers, and have a top speed of around 7 kph. However this is very limiting, as most treadmills have a top speed of 12 to 16 kph. Even if you don't intend to run, consider other family members who may use your machine, and the re-sale value. Also check out how quickly the buttons respond to changes when they are pressed. You don't want a slow response from the moving belt when you need to slow down or speed up the machine.
Cushioning	Some models will list shock absorption as a feature, which can reduce the stress on your feet, ankles and knees. If you have any lower leg problems, or if you intend to run occasionally, it is a feature well worth considering.
Noise	All treadmills make noise, but if you intend to watch TV or listen to music while exercising, make sure you can hear yourself think. Loud noise can reflect a less than powerful motor being pushed to its limit.
Safety features	Some treadmills have an emergency shut-off system that is very useful, especially for beginners or fast runners. The system usually involves a magnetic key on a chord which is clipped on to the clothes of the user. If the user falls or goes too far back on the belt, the magnetic key is pulled off and the treadmill will stop operating. Some machines also have an emergency stop button prominently displayed.

Belt width and thickness	Some treadmills have a very narrow belt, especially the cheaper models. This can limit your movement and even be dangerous. Always try before you buy, and make sure the belt width is wide enough to make you feel comfortable. Also, check the belt thickness for quality, as some cheaper versions curl up at the edge and form a tripping hazard.
Heart rate monitoring	Some treadmills have receivers for a heart rate monitor chest strap, or hand sensors that you hold for a few seconds for a read out of your heart rate. Avoid ear clip heart rate monitors, as they are extremely inaccurate. If this is something you value, you can always purchase a monitor separately for outdoor use as well.
Display console	The typical console will display your speed, incline, time, distance and kilojoules burned. Additional features could include pace, lap time, preset speed buttons, heart rate, CD player, drink holder and a reading ledge. Make sure the numbers are easy to read.
Folding versus fixed	Foldable treadmills are useful if space is a concern. Just make sure that there is no loss of stability. Also check how safe the latch mechanism is that holds the treadmill in the folded position, especially if you have small children.
Stability	It's important that the treadmill is stable while you walk on it, especially at higher inclines. Cheaper models may rock backwards and forth, or from side to side, making you feel insecure.
Price	Set a budget for how much you wish to spend. Prices start from around $1500, and can go upwards of several thousand dollars. If you can't find what you want, consider second hand models, ex-rentals, or save up till you can afford the model you want.
After sales service	Find out about what kind of warranty you get with the treadmill, and how accessible replacement parts are. I can speak from experience in saying that things do go wrong with electronic/ computerised fitness equipment.
Programs	Many machines have pre-programmed features that automatically adjust the speed/ and/or incline while you walk or run. Some even allow you to customise and pre-program your own workouts. These features are accessible through the display console, and can add interest and variety over the long term.
Others	Drink holders may not seem important, but they will keep you on your treadmill longer. Also check the handrail location. You don't want to hit your hands when you swing your arms. Finally, make sure you are comfortable with the deck size, which is the length of the walking surface.

Trainer's tip – No motor, no deal

Steer clear of un-motorised treadmills. While they are cheap, they are much less effective at fat burning because you can't swing your arms. They can also injure your back.

To rent or buy

If you are unsure about what treadmill to buy or whether you will really use it enough, why not try hiring one for a few months. You will see how much value you would get out of the machine at a fraction of the cost. Some companies even have a hire/buy scheme, where the rental price comes off the purchase price should you decide you wish to own it. I even have some clients who just hire a treadmill every winter. Just look up exercise equipment in your local *Yellow Pages* to find your nearest supplier.

12

Stretching and injury prevention

General stretching guidelines

To help maximise the effectiveness of your stretching, incorporate these 3 phases into your routine, performed one after the other.

1. **Ease in** – Gradually move into a light stretch and hold until the feeling of tension begins to diminish (usually after 5 to 10 seconds).

2. **The development** – Now, move a fraction further into the stretch until you feel mild tension again. Don't let the stretch become painful. Hold for another 5 to 10 seconds, then slowly ease out of the stretch. This technique really helps to loosen muscles and reduce tension.

3. **Repeat** – It is also beneficial to repeat phase 1 and 2 after backing out of the stretch for a few seconds.

Guidelines for safe and effective stretching

- Ease gradually in and out of each stretch
- Avoiding bouncing, jerky movements
- Don't stretch cold muscles
- Don't stretch to the point of pain
- Stretch immediately after exercise
- Stretch at least 3 times per week for the best results
- Don't compare your level of stretching with others
- Hold stretches for at least 10 to 20 seconds

Stretches for walkers

The most important muscles to stretch are those used predominantly for walking. These include the muscles of the front and back of your thighs, your calves, and your buttocks. Apply the general stretching guidelines to these specific stretches.

- **Stretch your thighs** – To stretch your quadriceps (the group of muscles in the front of your thighs) stand on one foot and hold on to a wall or solid object for balance. Reach behind your back and grab the foot of your free hanging leg, pulling your heel towards your bottom. Pull it in gently until you feel tension in the muscles in the front of your thigh. If your heel actually touches your bottom and you don't feel a stretch, make sure you are standing up straight, that the knee of the leg being stretched is behind the knee of the leg you are standing on, that your hips are slightly forward, and your shoulders are slightly back. Repeat with the opposite leg.

- **Stretch your buttocks** – Lie on your back with your knees bent at approximately 90 degrees. Keep your right foot on the ground at this stage, and rest your left ankle on your right thigh, just above your knee. Bring your right thigh towards you, and grab it with both hands. Your left hand should reach through your legs, while your right hand can grab the back of your right thigh from the side. Gently pull the right thigh towards you, which will also pull your left ankle closer to you, and begin to stretch your left buttock. Repeat with the opposite leg.

- **Stretch your inner thighs (groin)** – Sit on the floor and bring the soles of your feet in together towards your buttocks so they are touching. Slowly press your knees towards the floor while keeping your back straight. If you don't feel the stretch, lean forwards a little and push down a little harder on your knees.

- **Stretch your calf** – Stand facing a wall or solid object, placing both hands up against it, and reach one leg back behind you. Keep the heel of your back foot on the ground and your rear leg straight as you lean forwards towards the wall. Keep your back straight and your abdominal muscles tight. If you don't feel the stretch, move your hands lower, and place your foot further back behind you. Repeat with the other leg.

  Variation – *Perform exactly the same stretch, except bend your back knee. This will help to target your lower calf and Achilles tendon.*

- **Stretch your hamstrings** – Stand on one leg and place the other leg straight out in front of you on top of a table, chair or other stable object. The outstretched leg should be close to parallel with the ground. Gently bend forward and slide your hands towards the elevated foot until you begin to feel the stretch behind your knee. Repeat on your other leg.

  Variation – *Perform the same stretch, but bend the knee of your outstretched leg slightly. This will stretch the higher portion of your hamstrings (closer to your buttocks).*

Injury prevention

Isn't walking safe?

While walking is a low-impact activity, it's important to stay injury free if you are going to get results. Your feet have to endure an average of 5000 to 10 000 steps a day (even more if you are active). That's a lot of force that your feet, ankles, knees, hips and back have to absorb, so things are bound to go wrong occasionally. But a few simple steps can make all the difference when it comes to reducing your risk of injury and increasing the safety of your walking routine. I have already discussed the importance of warming up in Chapter 5. Following are some strategies you can use to keep your walking footloose and trouble free.

Don't go too hard too early

If you have been inactive for some time, ease yourself into your new walking program. Start out at a level where you feel comfortable. Train at a low intensity for 2 to 4 weeks so your muscles and ligaments can adjust to your increased level of activity. This will help prepare your body for the specific stresses and movement involved in walking. Over the longer term, you will get the best results by gradually pushing yourself a little further or faster each workout, and not going like a bull at a gate from the start. Focus on where you will be in 2 months, not in 2 weeks.

Warm up first

A warm up increases circulation and helps to prepare your muscles for exercise, making them more flexible and less likely to tear or strain. This is especially important if you haven't exercised in some time. Because walking is a low-intensity activity, it's not important to perform any extra exercises or stretches. Just start at a slower speed for the first 2 to 3 minutes of your walk. This low intensity movement will gradually increase your heart rate using the specific muscles that are used during walking. As your walking speed improves, or if you are already walking fast, you will need to warm up for longer. One useful guide is to exercise at a lower intensity until your heart rate reaches 100 beats per minute.

Stop if something's not right

If you feel any pain, discomfort or dizziness during your walks, stop immediately. If the pain doesn't stop, or if the pain was severe, seek medical attention. If the pain stops, resume walking at a lower level or intensity. Try to identify the specific nature and location of your pain and how far into your walk you were before the pain occurred. It may help to look at the common injuries that occur in walkers later in this chapter, and see if any of these relate to the pain you experienced. Don't feel that you need to walk through pain. You may experience a little discomfort when starting out, but 'no pain, no gain' is a complete myth in relation to weight loss. Only more advanced or elite walkers need to push to the point of pain, but they should also be fit enough to tolerate training at a higher level of exertion.

Cool down after your walk

At the end of your walk, reduce your speed to cool down your body. Try to cool down for 5 to 10 minutes to help your body to adjust from an active state to a resting state. Try to avoid a sudden stop to your walk, which can cause dizziness, soreness and cramps. By keeping your body moving, your muscles contract helping to pump blood back to the heart. If you are a beginner, and your walks are short, you only need to cool down for a minute or two. As your walking time and intensity increases, so should your cool-down period afterwards.

Stretch afterwards

Stretching helps to realign muscles that are used and shortened during walking. It can improve your athletic performance, prevent injury and soreness, and increase the enjoyment of your exercise routine. Walking is a low-intensity activity, so it's not necessary to stretch beforehand. But it will be beneficial for you to take the time to stretch after every workout.

Walking in the heat

Preparation is the key to enjoying your walks and other activities during the warmer months. To prevent heat-induced illness, consider the following tips.

- **Drink plenty of water** – Make sure you drink before, during and after walking in the heat. Don't wait till you're thirsty, as you may already be partially dehydrated. Little sips of cool water are best, while sports drinks are helpful if your activity is longer than 60 minutes.
- **Know the symptoms of dehydration** – Early signs of dehydration include thirst, light-headedness, tiredness, grogginess, nausea and a cold, clammy feeling. If these warning signs are ignored, more serious symptoms may develop, including heat cramps, heat exhaustion and heat stroke.
- **Sun protection** – Follow the normal rules of sun care, such as wearing a hat or cap, an appropriate shirt, and use 30+ sunscreen. Make sure to apply cream to danger areas such as your face, neck, the tips of your ears and the back of your hands. If you are sweating heavily, you may need to re-apply sunscreen.

- **Schedule your walks wisely** – Try to plan your walks or activities early in the morning or later in the evening, when the humidity and temperature is lower. Try to stay in the shade where possible, and avoid the sun when it's strongest.
- **Take a break** – If you go for longer walks, it might be wise to include a few rest breaks in the extreme heat. You might even consider shorter walks, or opt for a water-based activity if it's too hot.

Walking in the cold

There is usually no reason why you can't continue to walk in the colder months, provided the weather isn't extreme. Being a little cold while you walk will actually help to increase your kilojoule use and fat burning capacity. Chapter 5 discussed the most appropriate clothing for walking in cold weather. Following are some additional tips to ensure your walks are safe and enjoyable.

- **Do a longer warm up** – Start a little slower than normal, and gradually ease your body into your walk. Cold weather requires you to warm up for longer.
- **Keep your fluid levels up** – Cold weather stimulates urine production, and with every breath you can see water droplets being exhaled from your body. Drinking water regularly is just as important during cold weather as it is in warm weather.
- **Rug up against the wind** – Wind can significantly increase heat loss from your body. Cold air that is moving at speed can be colder than just normal air temperature, and is known as the 'wind chill factor'. If it is windy outside, consider additional layers, gloves, headwear and appropriate wind-proof clothing.
- **Communicate with your doctor** – Some medical conditions make winter exercise dangerous. Exercising in cold weather can bring on angina (heart-related chest pain), and may trigger asthma in asthmatics. Check first with your doctor if you have any concerns, especially if you are older or have been sedentary for more than 2 months.

Walking in darkness

If you walk in the evening or early morning, it's important to wear brightly coloured clothing to increase your visibility. Reflective strips or panels are also available on some shoes and clothing. If there are no footpaths where you are, walk facing the traffic, which helps you identify any possible danger coming towards you. Try to anticipate the most likely actions drivers will take, and expect them not to see you. If you have any personal safety concerns, look for well-lit paths, and try to walk with someone else, or even a dog. You can also carry a torch, whistle or personal alarm.

Common problems and their treatment

Blisters

Blisters are caused by friction, and are one of the most common ailments affecting walkers and runners. To prevent blisters, wear correctly fitting shoes, use thick absorbent socks, and apply petroleum jelly, sports tape or talcum powder on the areas that generally blister. Treatment for a blister depends on its size. Smaller blisters can be left alone or covered with a Band-Aid. For larger blisters, clean the area first with an antibacterial ointment, and puncture it with a sterile lance or needle to drain the liquid. The hole should be large enough so the liquid can drain, but small enough so that skin remains to protect the soft under-layer of skin. To reduce the risk of infection, cover the area with a Band-Aid and keep your foot as dry as possible.

Chafing

Chafing commonly occurs on the inner thigh and groin area due to friction from clothing or body parts rubbing together. It can also occur on the nipples of both men and women, and can be very painful. To prevent chafing, try to stay dry, drink plenty of water, and wear the proper clothing such as bike pants, or clothes with minimal flat seams. You can apply talcum powder to stay dry, or a lubricant like petroleum jelly to prevent friction. To treat chafing, wash the area with lukewarm water, and apply an antibacterial ointment to prevent infection. You can also cover the chafing with a sterile gauze pad that gives protection, but still promotes healing by allowing the area to breathe.

Muscle cramps

Muscle cramps are painful, unpredictable, involuntary muscle contractions that can affect anyone during exercise. Although cramps may occasionally be the result of fluid and electrolyte (sodium) imbalance from sweating, that is not usually the case. A recent study showed that contrary to popular belief, cramps are not usually caused by dehydration, blocked blood flow, nerve damage, or electrolyte abnormalities of calcium, sodium, magnesium or potassium. The researchers showed that the most likely cause is muscle fatigue. Cramps are most common when you use your muscles beyond their normal limits. You can prevent muscle cramps by warming up and cooling down when exercising, staying well hydrated, and conditioning yourself for your chosen activity. To treat a muscle cramp, stop your activity and stretch the affected muscle.

General soreness after walking

When you first commence, return to, or reinvigorate an exercise program, it's normal to experience muscle soreness within 12 to 48 hours of your activity. You may also experience a little muscle stiffness and fatigue. This is how your muscles adapt to the new stresses being placed upon them. It can last for the first 1 to 3 weeks of your program, after which you should experience minimal if any soreness after exercise. To prevent this delayed muscle soreness, warm up, cool down, stretch afterwards and commence your program gradually. To treat muscle soreness, do some low-intensity exercise, stretch the specific area, get a massage, or rest if the pain is intense. If the pain doesn't dissipate after 3 to 5 days, seek medical attention.

Shin splints

A shin splint is a general term used to describe overuse injuries common amongst walkers and runners from frequent activity on non-resilient surfaces like concrete. Constant jarring can lead to micro-trauma and small muscle tears where the calf muscle attaches to your shin, resulting in pain up the front of your leg. It can also relate to stress reactions along the long bones of your shin. To prevent shin splints, strengthen and stretch the muscles of your lower leg, and try to choose softer surfaces to exercise on. If the pain from your shin splints is minor, cut back your workload a little, stretch the affected area and apply ice. If the pain occurs during exercise and is limiting your performance, you may need complete rest, massage and cross training until the injury repairs. If you are a long-term sufferer, it may help to get a biomechanical analysis of your posture and gait, and professionally fitted shoes.

Side stitch

A side stitch is usually experienced as a pain just below the rib cage on the right side that occurs during exercise. It's thought this pain is caused by a stretching of the ligaments that extend from your diaphragm to the internal organs, particularly the liver. People who exhale when their right foot hits the ground (about 30 per cent of people) force the liver to go down as their diaphragm goes up during breathing. This stretches the ligaments in between and causes pain. People who breathe out when their left foot hits the ground are much less likely to get a side stitch. You can also prevent a side stitch by taking even, deep breaths while you run or walk, and avoid eating before exercise if you are vulnerable. To treat a stitch, stop your activity, then bend forward and tighten your abdominal muscles while breathing out through pursed lips. This is thought to reduce tension on the ligaments.

13

Walking and your health

Walking can do more for your health than just help you lose fat and weight. Some of the most common diseases and illnesses affecting Australians can be treated and prevented by walking regularly.

Walking for your heart

In Australia, 1 in 2 people will die prematurely from heart disease. Although a heart attack can be sudden, it usually reflects years of poor lifestyle habits. Inactivity is well established as a major risk factor for heart disease, rating alongside smoking and high blood pressure. Conversely, walking speeds up the circulation of blood around your body, helping the heart work more effectively and lowering blood pressure. In fact, regular walking can help to reduce the need for blood pressure medication. Walking can also help to lower LDL (bad) cholesterol and raise HDL (good) cholesterol. The greatest potential for the heart health benefits of exercise is in those who are least active, and the most suitable form of exercise for people who are inactive is walking.

Science says – Walk for your heart

Women who walked at least 3 hours per week had a 40 per cent lower risk of heart attack and stroke than sedentary women. Those who walked at a brisk pace had an even greater risk reduction (54 per cent).

What if I have an existing heart condition?

Many people with heart disease are timid about exercise, worrying that they might have a heart attack, or worsen their symptoms. Yet it only takes a few weeks of moderate walking to notice an improvement. Walking has even been shown to reverse some aspects of heart disease, such as restoring the elasticity of arteries. If you have an existing heart condition, your doctor will make recommendations for your exercise program based on your condition and stage of recovery. Walking is often recommended as an easy way to begin a physical activity program because it is such a low-intensity activity.

Science says – Mild exercise cuts heart deaths

Gentle exercise such as walking has been shown to cut death rates in cardiovascular patients by more than a third. Anyone who has ongoing cardiovascular problems would benefit greatly by walking regularly.

Heart health walking guidelines

Aim for 30 minutes of mild-intensity walking every day, or a little longer if you miss a day or two.

WARNING – Some heart patients may be at a stage where exercise is not recommended, so make sure you consult with your doctor.

Walking and arthritis

Unfortunately, more than 2 million Australians are familiar with the joint pain, inflammation and stiffness that comes with arthritis. Inflammation occurs for a number of reasons including injury, disease, infection, or merely the wear and tear that naturally occurs over time.

Exercises that build up your stamina, such as walking, help to reduce body fat, which can help to lower body weight and relieve pain. Walking can also help arthritis sufferers with pain management, provided the exercise program is individually tailored and combined with an appropriate amount of rest and recovery time.

Benefits from walking for arthritis sufferers

- Stronger muscles and bones
- Increased flexibility and stamina
- Improved sense of wellbeing and positive attitude
- Decreased pain
- Maintenance and improvement of joint movement
- Increased heart and lung fitness
- Improved posture
- Weight control
- Improved sleep patterns

Arthritis walking guidelines

Aim for 30 minutes of mild-intensity walking every day, or a little longer if you miss a day or two. While walking can reduce pain and help maintain joint flexibility, it should not be carried out during acutely painful phases of the disease.

Walking and diabetes

It's estimated that over 1 million Australians have diabetes, although only half that amount have actually been diagnosed. There are 3 main types of diabetes, all of which have different causes, and they can all be alleviated by regular walking. The three types of diabetes are:

- **Type 1 diabetes** – Previously known as 'insulin-dependent' or 'juvenile onset' diabetes, this is usually inherited.

- **Type 2 diabetes** – Previously known as 'non insulin-dependent' or 'adult onset' diabetes, this is the most common form of diabetes (85 per cent). It is usually triggered later in life as increasing body fat levels cause your body to resist insulin.

- **Gestational diabetes** – This type of diabetes only occurs in women who are pregnant, but it can predispose women to type 2 diabetes later in life.

The aim of all diabetes management is to keep blood sugar levels within the normal range. Walking can protect against all types of diabetes because it helps to lower and stabilise blood sugar levels. It also helps to keep your level of body fat down, which increases the effectiveness of insulin. Ultimately, walking can not only help to treat all types of diabetes, it can help to prevent type 2 and gestational diabetes as well.

Diabetes walking guidelines

Aim for 30 minutes of mild-intensity walking every day, or a little longer if you miss a day or two. Diabetics should not follow the advice to walk before breakfast, or delay eating after exercise to maximise fat burning. This could lead to hyperglycaemia, where blood sugar levels become dangerously low.

WARNING – If your blood sugar control is poor, or if you have diabetic eye disease, it's best to seek medical advice before you start a new exercise program. If you have type 1 diabetes, you may also want to discuss any changes to how much insulin you need, as exercise can alter this.

Mental health

We've all have bad days when we feel down and in a bad mood. But if that bad mood never goes away, you may be suffering from depression, thought to affect 1 in 5 people from all age groups, social classes and ethnic backgrounds. You are more than likely to experience mental illness at some point in your life, either directly or through a friend or family member. A lack of public knowledge and understanding about depression makes it difficult for sufferers and their families to even acknowledge there is a problem or seek treatment. Unfortunately, many people view depression as a sign of weakness rather than a treatable illness. However, appropriate treatment can help over 80 per cent of sufferers. Treatment usually involves medication, psychotherapy and lifestyle changes. Physical activity has been prescribed for the treatment of depression, with research showing it to be as effective as standard drug therapy in reducing symptoms. People who walked briskly for 30 minutes reported an improved mood for up to an hour after their workout. People who exercise regularly are also less likely to become depressed.

How walking can help relieve depression

- Relieves muscle tension
- Boosts alertness and heart rate
- Encourages relaxation and sleep
- Provides a safe outlet for frustration
- Boosts energy levels
- Improves self-esteem
- Changes the focus of your mind towards a repetitive, meditative activity

Depression walking guidelines

Aim for 30 minutes of mild-intensity walking every day, or a little longer if you miss a day or two. Consistent walking together with medication and counselling can help people treat, manage and overcome depression.

WARNING – For some people, exercise alone will not eliminate all the symptoms of mental illness. Medication is often necessary to correct chemical imbalances in the brain for severe depression or anxiety. Do not alter your level of medication without consulting a specialist. If you experience any of the symptoms of depression, such as feelings of hopelessness, worthlessness or helplessness, loss of interest in the things that used to give you pleasure or suicidal thoughts, it's important you consult a mental health specialist.

Walking and asthma

Australia has one of the highest rates of asthma in the world. Fortunately, asthmatics can use exercise to their advantage, because it can improve cardiovascular fitness and help to manage the condition. The fitter an asthmatic is the easier it is for their lungs to expel air, and the less breathing will be needed for a given amount of exercise. Due to its rhythmic, continuous nature, walking is much less likely to provoke an asthma attack than a high-intensity workout. Most asthmatics experience a narrowing of the airways during exercise, especially with strenuous activity in cold, dry air. But this can be relieved with bronchodilators, such as Ventolin, which quickly open up constricted airways.

Science says – Body fat linked to asthma

Obesity may increase the risk of developing asthma in adulthood, especially in women. A study of over 89 000 women aged 27 to 41 found that as their level of body fat increased, so did their risk of developing asthma. The risk for adult-onset asthma was almost three times higher in clinically obese women compared with women in the healthy weight range. It's thought that excess body fat may compress the lungs, increasing bronchial reactivity. It's another good reason to walk off weight.

Asthma walking guidelines

Aim for 30 minutes of mild intensity walking every day, or a little longer if you miss a day or two. When overall control of asthma is good, the symptoms of exercise-induced asthma are unlikely to be a problem. But there are some strategies that can help to prevent an attack.

- Take a normal dose of a bronchodilator immediately prior to your walk.
- Take your medication with you during your walk.
- Always warm up before walking to relax the chest muscles and widen the airways.
- Reduce your pace and duration during cold weather, and when pollution or pollen counts are high.
- Stay well hydrated during your walks.
- Perform nasal breathing where possible to increase the moisture and humidity of the air.

WARNING – While walking can be beneficial for asthmatics, it can also trigger an attack. Work closely with your doctor to establish an asthma management plan designed to control the symptoms of asthma. By using preventative strategies and medication as needed, most people with exercise-induced asthma can participate in walking safely and enjoyably.

Walking and bone health

Osteoporosis involves the gradual weakening of bones, especially among women over 50. Unfortunately, osteoporosis is becoming more common in younger men and women. It is a silent disease with no symptoms. The only warning sign that your bones have become weaker is from a bone density scan, or from a fracture. Fortunately, walking is known to decrease bone loss, increase bone density, and reduce the risk of fractures. Walking is a weight-bearing exercise, where the weight of your body is transmitted through the bones as they work against gravity. Your bones respond to this force by growing stronger.

Science says – Walking promotes bone density

A recent study on women compared one group who walked for 30 minutes 3 times a week with a group of sedentary women over a 4-month period. The women who walked gained close to 0.4 per cent in bone mineral density in the lower spine, while the sedentary women saw a decrease of nearly 2 per cent. Walkers also saw a 1.4 per cent gain in the thighbone, while the non-walkers lost about 0.6 per cent.

Bone health walking guidelines

Aim for 30 to 45 minutes of mild-intensity walking every day, or a little longer if you miss a day or two. Consistency is important, as you need to keep putting the weight-bearing stress on your bones to maintain the extra bone density you have gained.

WARNING – If you have been diagnosed with osteoporosis, avoid high impact activities during your walks, such as jogging. This can cause too much jarring of the spine, and can increase the risk of vertebral fractures.

Walking and sexual health

There is an important relationship between your overall health and sexual satisfaction. For men, impotence can be an early warning sign of heart and artery disease due to a reduction in blood flow. Exercise such as walking is known to improve circulation, promoting blood flow and helping to minimise blood vessel blockages. Walking can improve a host of women's sexual health issues, including mood and libido. Cardiovascular fitness can boost your stamina and your appearance, which are both important for sexual performance and confidence.

Science says – Walking instead of Viagra

A 9-year study on 600 men found that a brisk 30-minute walk each day can reduce a man's risk of developing impotence. Exercise was shown to keep the blood flowing and prevent impotence in the same way it prevents heart attacks.

Walking and sexual health guidelines

Aim for 30 minutes of walking every day for maximum sexual health benefits. Jogging or other activities that burn around 800 kilojoules and increase the heart rate are also said to be beneficial.

Walking and longevity

Physical activity and its side effect of weight management are both proven to improve the quality and quantity of life. Walking is proven to add many disease-free years to your life, and has a wide range of health benefits and anti-ageing effects. These include lower blood pressure and blood fats, protection against diabetes and obesity, and improved balance, which helps prevents fracture-causing falls. Exercise has been shown to reduce death rates, regardless of genetic makeup. A 20-year study on active twins who walked for 30 minutes 6 or more times a week found a 43 per cent reduced risk of dying compared to their couch potato sibling. Another study found that walking for 30 minutes a day lengthened a person's life by more than a year, and also added a year of life without heart disease compared to people with low activity levels. Even for the elderly, regular activity is less dangerous to your health than inactivity.

Science says – Lose fat to live longer

Recent studies have shown that obesity can cut more than 10 years from a person's lifespan. Obesity is particularly dangerous for younger adults, and is a well-known risk factor for heart disease, diabetes and other chronic diseases that can cause premature death. Another study showed that middle-aged subjects who walked briskly cut their heart disease risk in half, whether or not they exercised when they were young.

Walking and longevity guidelines

Aim for 30 minutes 6 or more times a week for maximum longevity effects. However, people who do any exercise still have a lower mortality risk compared to those who don't exercise at all.

14

Walking for kids

Children's health is in crisis

One in 4 Australian kids is overweight or obese. The cause is a combination of high-kilojoule, junk food-rich diets and low levels of intentional and incidental activity. As body fat levels increase, so does the risk of developing a number of illness and diseases that can dramatically reduce life quality and quantity. There are also social pressures and self-esteem issues associated with being an overweight child.

 Science says – Growing out, not up

> Studies have shown that approximately 60 per cent of obese children become obese adults. Many of these obese children will also develop diabetes at a young age.

What can parents do?

The alarming statistics on childhood weight and obesity should only serve to increase our sense of urgency in taking action, yet very little has been done. It's no surprise to learn that young Australians are less active than ever before. However, regular physical activity must be a major priority for children of all ages. Parents have an important role to play. Try to encourage your kids to be active from an early age to help them develop and function optimally both physically and mentally. This can help to boost their self-esteem and foster a positive lifelong attitude towards activity, exercise and sport. It also helps to discourage inactive pastimes like television viewing and computer games.

How can walking help?

Walking is not only one of the best exercises to treat a childhood weight problem, it can also help to prevent it. It's inexpensive, requires no coordination or equipment, and can be done anywhere. Walking more is the first step in finding a long-term cure for motion deprivation and couch potato disease. Because virtually anyone can walk, it creates a positive connection between physical activity and achievement. Exercise doesn't have to involve sweat, discomfort or pain to benefit your child. Walking can be fun and adventurous for children, which creates a link between physical activity and enjoyment. These underlying connections with achievement and enjoyment through walking can potentially encourage kids to try other activities, and develop a positive attitude towards physical activity for the rest of their lives.

Science says – Preventing weight gain in children

A new study discovered walking 2000 extra daily steps (which can be measured with a pedometer) and cutting back 400 kilojoules each day can prevent weight gain in overweight children.

Get your kids to walk to school

Safety fears and expanding suburb boundaries have resulted in most kids sitting down in a bus or car on the way to school instead of walking. But encouraging your children to walk to school will have many positive benefits for their health and development. Depending on your child's age, they can walk with you, walk themselves (if over the age of 10), walk part of the way if you drive them part of the way, or walk with other children. They will arrive at school alert and attentive, and learn how to incorporate physical activity into their everyday lives. Some schools have even started a program where kids walk together, sing, play musical instruments and walk puppies. Others have a walking bus, where a parent or teacher supervises a group who walks a set route and picks up children along the way. They interact with other children in a fun way, and get some exercise in before arriving at school. Maybe you could investigate the possibility of developing such initiatives at your child's school.

Make walking to school safe for your child

- Walk with your child until they develop a good sense of road safety, especially at road crossings.
- Arrange adult supervision, or accompany your child until the age of 10.
- Show them the safest path with the least amount of traffic and road crossings.
- Teach them to use the footpath instead of the road wherever possible.

- Encourage them not to play with balls or other toys as they walk.
- Encourage them not to use portable music devices, or at least keep the volume low so they can hear traffic.
- Teach them to be aware of cars coming in and out of driveways.
- Get them to walk with other children if you have concerns about safety.
- Make them aware of safety houses with up-to-date registration – places they can go along the way if they feel threatened by strangers or bullies.

Be a role model

As a parent, your knowledge of nutrition, the foods you provide, the example that you set and your attitude towards exercise will affect the health of your child. By setting a good example, parents have a unique opportunity to be a positive influence on their children's eating and activity habits. Children are good learners, and they learn by what they see. It's a classic case of monkey see, monkey do. Choose healthy foods and active pursuits for yourself. Don't tell your child to go outside and play while you eat chips on the couch. The best method is to change the whole family's approach to diet and encourage all family members to be more active. This benefits everyone, and doesn't single out overweight children.

Walk on weekends

Your child's health will benefit from any activity that takes them away from watching television and DVDs, playing console games or surfing the internet. These inactive pastimes are the most common form of entertainment for many children, and significantly reduce their opportunities to be active. But don't force your kids to exercise. Try to incorporate walking into your family activities, such as picnics, bushwalks and trips to the beach. Walking with your children on weekends or on holidays is a great way to enjoy quality time with them. You can take the dog, go the park and play, get something you need at the shops, or visit friends or family.

Slim trim & tasty

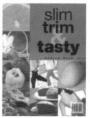

By Andrew Cate

(Food styling by Donna Hay)

Andrew's first book combines 40 pages of fat loss information with tasty, healthy recipes to help you lose body fat. The book includes quizzes, tips, quotes and a fat and fibre counter. You will also find more than 60 recipes, most of which are pictured in colour, with each one's fat and fibre content per serving. Many of the recipes have been selected to provide choices that are not traditionally associated with a healthy diet—Choccy mud muffins, Macaroni cheese, Pizza, Cheesy fish fillets, Carrot and Banana cakes, Hummus, San choy bow, French onion dip.

Only $15 posted anywhere in Australia.
Visit www.andrewcate.com for more information.

Ask the Fat Loss Coach

101 questions answered about food, fitness and fat loss

By Andrew Cate

This ebook tells you everything you have ever wanted to know about removing stored body fat. Andrew has spent 15 years in the fitness industry, so he knows the answers to some of the most frequently asked questions relating to health, fitness, nutrition and fat loss. The book is written in Andrew's easy-to-read style, and has plenty of tables, quotes and practical tips. Some of the questions he answers include 'Should you have a junk food day?', 'Is swimming a good fat loss exercise?', 'Am I getting enough iron?', 'Can you help me with my New Year's resolutions?' and 'What exercise machine is most likely to help me get results?' **Emailed to you for just $10, or sent to you on disk for $15.**
Visit www.andrewcate.com for more information.

- ✂

YOUR ORDER

☐ Slim Trim & Tasty $15
☐ Ask the Fat Loss Coach—email $10
☐ Ask the Fat Loss Coach—disk $15

              Your Total   [   ]

PAYMENT

☐ BPay: Biller Code: 1008   Reference Number: 4557 0256 6937 3736
Email your receipt number, name, address and phone number to: acate@iprimus.com.au

☐ Cheque   ☐ Money Order   (Cheques or Money Orders payable to 'Andrew Cate')

DETAILS

Name: _____   Phone Day: (____) _____

Address:_____ Suburb:_____

P/code:_____   Email:_____

Provide the details above with your payment by post or email to receive your order.

Send to: Andrew Cate, 13A Waterview St, Mona Vale NSW 2103,
or email: acate@iprimus.com.au